Mental Health Approaches to Intellectual/Developmental Disability:
A Resource for Trainers

Robert J. Fletcher, DSW, ACSW, NADD-CC
Daniel Baker, PhD, NADD-CC
Juanita St Croix, BSc
Melissa Cheplic, MPH

Table of Contents

Introduction

Welcome to *Mental Health Approaches to Intellectual/Developmental Disability: A Resource for Trainers*. This is a landmark contribution to the field of support for persons with Intellectual or Developmental Disabilities (IDD) and Mental Health concerns. This Resource for Trainers can be used by a myriad of different professionals and care providers for a variety of different purposes. *Mental Health Approaches to Intellectual/ Developmental Disability: A Resource for Trainers* may be used: (a) to train others for professional development (train-the-trainer model), (b) as a resource guide for individual study, or (c) as a reference guide. Proper support of mental wellness among persons with IDD requires a significant body of information and knowledge, and the authors of this Resource for Trainers are happy to offer it as a means for educating professionals and care providers. The overall mission of this Resource for Trainers is to provide an overview of mental health concerns and support for persons with IDD.

This Resource for Trainers is designed to be used with a wide variety of audiences – from advanced professionals, who may not have specific training in this area, to Direct Support Professionals. As such, the material was selected to have a base level of information for the learner, with more content introduced as appropriate. For professionals seeking a more advanced level of information, citations have been provided at the end of each module. Additionally, more advanced materials can be found via The NADD Press.

Trainers often have the challenge of working with sessions' attendees with disparate experience. Skilled trainers and teachers can provide different levels of engagement to different attendees, differentiating instruction by asking different questions and providing leadership roles in small group activities for more experienced attendees. Lecture notes in this Resource for Trainers often contain content which can be used at the trainer's discretion.

This Resource for Trainers includes printed materials and a flash drive containing PowerPoint slides for use in training on this material. The Manual is printed in black and white, but the flash drive is in full digital color.

The Resource for Trainers is organized into modules. Each module begins with learning objectives. Within the module, materials are presented in Microsoft PowerPoint, with slides and Speaker's Notes.

Using the Resource for Trainers to Train Others for Professional Development

Use the enclosed flash drive to access the MS PowerPoint files. The Speaker's Notes are to be used as a resource for you as you engage in the training. PowerPoint's "Presenter view" enables you to view speaker notes on one computer monitor while the audience views the notes-free presentation on a different monitor. PowerPoint's help provides directions for setting up "Presenter view." Exercises and Case Studies are included to give the attendees a chance to practice and interact with the materials being presented. Please refer to our Trainer's Tips section for further suggestions regarding conducting a training session.

A workbook, *Trainee Workbook for Mental Health Approaches to Intellectual/Developmental Disability,* is available and is intended to be used by participants in your trainings. It contains the slides (without Speaker's Notes) and space for the participant to write his or her own notes. The workbook contains pre-and post-tests for each module to measure and assist in learning. These pre- and post-tests are also included in the Appendix of the Resource for Trainers.

Using the Resource for Trainers for Individual Study

When used as a resource for individual study, we encourage reviewing and reading the entire Resource for Trainers. The material is comprehensive, and references are provided for further or more in-depth study as well as indicating original source material.

Using the Resource for Trainers as a Reference Guide

The organization of this Resource for Trainers is in a Module format, so if you have specific interest in any area, you can specifically review that topic.

About the Authors

Robert J. Fletcher, DSW, ACSW, NADD-CC

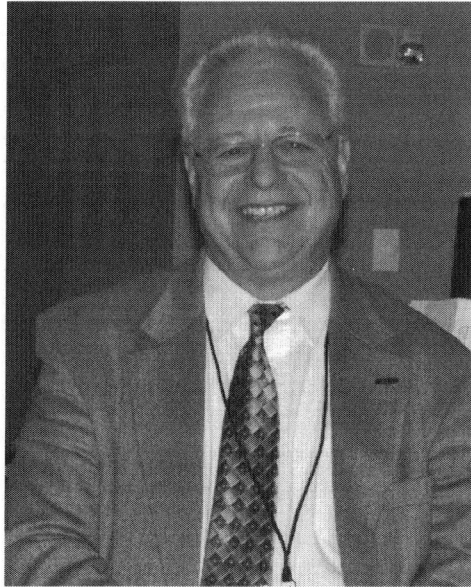

Robert J. Fletcher, DSW, ACSW, NADD-CC is the Founder and Chief Executive Officer of NADD. His vision and leadership have brought NADD to a position where it is recognized as the world's leading organization in providing educational resources, training materials, consultation services, and conferences concerning mental health aspects in persons with Intellectual Disabilities, as well as an accreditation/certification program.

Dr. Fletcher has dedicated his professional career to improving the lives of individuals who have a dual diagnosis of Mental Illness (MI) and an Intellectual Disability (ID). He has authored articles, book chapters, and books in areas concerning clinical, programmatic, policy and research in the field of dual diagnosis. He is the Chief Editor of both the textbook and clinical guide of the *Diagnostic Manual – Intellectual Disabilities (DM-ID)*. Most recently he has edited a book entitled *Psychotherapy for Individuals with Intellectual Disability*. Additionally, Dr. Fletcher provides consultation services and lectures on various topics related to mental health aspects in persons with Intellectual Disabilities.

Daniel Baker, PhD, NADD-CC

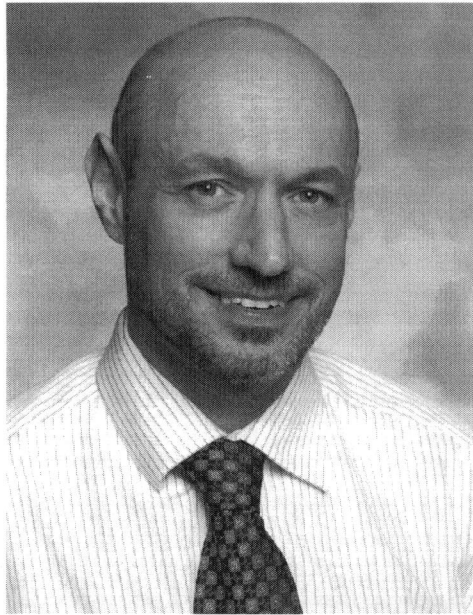

Dr. Dan Baker's focus at The Boggs Center is on positive behavior support, models of community and educational support, transition services, and mental health services for persons with disabilities. Dr. Baker earned his PhD in Educational Psychology in 1992 and a Teaching License in 1990 from the University of Minnesota. He has worked with people with a range of disabilities; his applied work includes efforts in schools, residential settings for people with disabilities, recreational programs, and employment supports.

Dr. Baker is well published in both edited books and literary journals. Most of his published work addresses strategies for teaching direct care staff to work with persons who present challenges. His contributions earned him the 2010 Clinical Practice Award from NADD, an international professional association dedicated to advancing mental wellness for persons with Intellectual or Developmental Disabilities. Dr. Baker is a reviewer for the journals *Intellectual and Developmental Disabilities, American Journal of Intellectual and Developmental Disabilities,* and *Research in Developmental Disabilities.* Dr. Baker is very involved with NADD, an association for persons with developmental disabilities and mental health needs, serving on the Board of Directors and co-editing *The NADD Bulletin* from 2006 - 2011.

Juanita St Croix, Specialized Services Facilitator

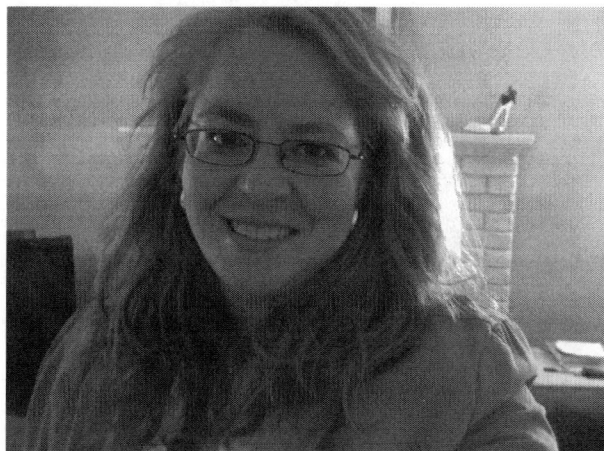

Juanita St Croix graduated Western University with a BSc. when it was still the University of Western Ontario. She has 22 years of experience in human services, primarily in developmental services with organizations providing services to people with complex behavioral support needs and a dual diagnosis.

Ms. St. Croix has been a facilitator with the Southern Network of Specialized Care since November 2010. Her work with the Network involves helping to build and support strong collaborative services for people who have a dual diagnosis, increasing the capacity of specialized clinical and direct support services in addressing the needs of people who have a dual diagnosis, and supporting research that also accomplishes these goals. With the Network, Ms. St Croix's work focuses significantly on research and publications.

Melissa Cheplic, MPH

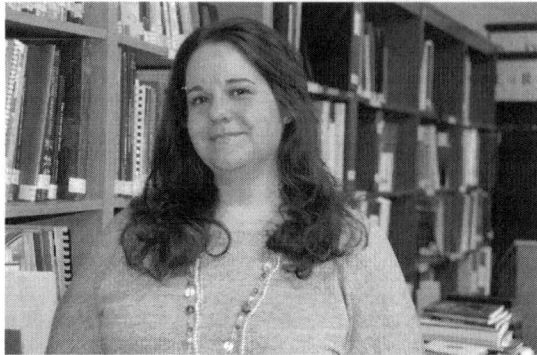

Melissa Cheplic is a Training and Consultation Specialist at *The Boggs Center on Developmental Disabilities at the Rutgers Robert Wood Johnson Medical School in New Jersey*. She works in the area of Positive Behavior Supports and Mental Health, developing and providing training and technical assistance to community support agencies and families. Ms. Cheplic has worked in the field as a trainer, counselor, advocate, and behavior specialist for children and adults with intellectual disabilities. Melissa is the Chairperson of The NADD Direct Support Professional Certification Committee and has presented nationally in the areas of Positive Behavior Support, Dual Diagnosis, Mental Health, and Competency- Based Curriculum Development. Ms. Cheplic received a Bachelor of Science Degree from Montclair State University and earned her Master's Degree in Public Health from the University of Medicine and Dentistry of New Jersey.

Training Tips

A trainer's role is to facilitate learning by creating conditions that are more favorable and effective than independent learning. A trainer's role is to add value to the learning process. We offer these general tips for training, and we make specific recommendations for use of this Resource for Trainers. We recognize that many of you may be extremely skilled trainers, but we offer these suggestions.

Preparing:

- Do your homework and preparation. Review all of the material numerous times so that you are completely familiar with all of the content. Look up any terminology or information with which you are unfamiliar. The citations (which appear in the reference lists) are good sources of research for more information. Make sure you have competency addressing this material before training on it.
- Prepare additional notes to supplement that which is provided in the speaker's notes. This can help clarify concepts that may be new to you and provide additional guidance while you are addressing participants.
- Evaluation can also be a useful tool to help identify and needed changes in presentation style, material, time lines, set up, etc. Prepare and offer an evaluation to attendees at the end of the training session. Rather than offering a standard NADD evaluation form, we encourage you to use one that your employer already utilizes.
- Make a list of materials you will need to complete the training. Include materials such as a computer, projector, pointer, markers, a flipchart, or other tools.
- Plan some opening remarks and how you are going to outline the day for the participants. You will want to identify where the material is conducive for breaks and times of the breaks.
- There is too much material here to attempt to cover all of it in a single day. Identify which module or modules will be covered. If all ten modules are to be covered, plan to accomplish this over the course of several days.
- Prepare an outline/agenda for participants to give them an understanding of how the training will proceed.
- Set expectations for participants about appropriate times to ask questions and give feedback aside from those outlined directly within the materials. Establish parameters for keeping focused on the material in order to complete learning goals within the allotted timeframe.
- Depending on the size of the group, you may want to prepare an "ice-breaker" exercise during which each person introduces him- or herself.

- In a larger group, you may want to poll the group by asking pertinent questions that will give you an indication of how many people are familiar with different concepts you will cover in the training. You can use the Learning Objectives appearing at the beginning of each module as your list for this.
- Plan to arrive early so you can set up and get a sense of the room in which you are training. It also gives you adequate time to set up any equipment or materials you are using and find out how different features work to change slides. Test the technology you will be using, if you are using a laptop or LCD projector before attendees arrive.
- Consider establishing a "parking lot" for items that will be addressed outside the general presentation of material or need to be considered for the curriculum. Make sure the participants know that you are there to get them the answers or help them find the answers.

During training:
- Don't forget to introduce yourself to the group. Provide a brief career biography that will offer the group some background information on your credentials and expertise. Establishing your credibility is important, so make sure that the attendees know that you have real experience. Talking about your success with individuals you have supported is important. While this Resource for Trainers offers many Case Studies, providing your own clinical examples is an excellent way to make the training become more real for you, more real to the participants, and help you to make a personal connection.
- When presenting, ensure you are not only reading off the slides, but speaking directly to the group of participants. Engage them with questions and encourage dialogue from the participants. Many of them may have some experience with the topics being presented and can enhance other participant learning by sharing examples from their own practices. Engaging the group in discussion will also contribute toward a collaborative network that can connect outside the training to share expertise and suggestions around issues that arise in the participants' practices.
- Breaking the group into several discussion groups to discuss a particular topic and then report back to the full group is a good way to foster interest and engagement. Consider doing this at least once for each training session.
- Outline the learning goals for each section when you begin it. Summarize at the beginning of a section what will be covered and the objectives and at the end of a section what was covered.
- If a question arises that is being covered in a later portion of the training or may lead the training in a different direction, record it in the parking lot. Assure the participant that the issue will be addressed more thoroughly at a later time, but clarify specific points essential for the learner to move on. For

questions that lead off topic, ask the questioner to speak with you during a break or at the end of the day. This will provide you an opportunity to address the question without veering off topic.

- Review your parking lot items at regular intervals. Note any items that may have been addressed. Confirm whether or not the person who asked the question feels that it has been answered to their understanding.

- Speaker's notes provide a guide for presenters to help make additional key points that are not on the slides. They are not intended to be a script, but a tool to give the trainer more information about the content. When delivering information on a particular slide, use the notes to learn more about a topic and help answer participant questions. Remember, good preparation is essential, and the use of your own notes is encouraged.

- Keep an eye on the time. Make sure you take breaks as planned in your outline of your presentation. Learning is more effective for participants when breaks are regularly scheduled throughout the training. Feel free to adjust breaks times as dictated by participants and other environmental factors.

- When addressing participants, be sure to use person first language that is gender and culturally sensitive. Take care when using sarcasm, idioms, and other expressions that can be misconstrued.

After the training:
- Make sure you thank everyone for participating. Offer them suggestions on how to get more information on the topic if interested.

- Be available, if possible, for a limited period to continue the discussion informally, if time remains within the allotted period.

- Gather your equipment and materials. It is good practice to ensure you leave the training room in good condition. Pick up any materials/resources the participants have left.

- Review the post-training evaluations for tips on enhancing the training, evaluation of the materials, and general information. Try not to take negative evaluations personally and use them as opportunities to determine if the comments are valid or what may be the source of the issue. Every trainer has gotten some silly or mean evaluations. Always remember that the purpose of evaluation is improvement.

- When preparing for the next training, use the feedback from the evaluations to enhance your presentation of the materials as needed.

What Is a Dual Diagnosis?

Slide 1

Mental Health Approaches to
Intellectual/Developmental Disability:
A Resource for Trainers

Dr. Robert J. Fletcher
      Founder and CEO, NADD
Dr. Dan Baker
      The Boggs Center, Rutgers RWJMS
Juanita St.Croix,
      Regional Support Associates/The
      Southern Network of Specialized Care
Melissa Cheplic, MPH
      The Boggs Center, Rutgers RWJMS

Slide 2

Module I

What is a Dual Diagnosis?

MODULE I

Slide 3

CONCEPT OF DUAL DIAGNOSIS

The concept of dual diagnosis was coined by the late Frank J. Menolascino, MD. (Menolascino, 1977)

The term is used in two different ways: (1) mental illness/substance abuse (MI/CA); (2) intellectual/developmental disability/mental illness (IDD/MI). However, in this context, the term dual diagnosis refers to IDD co-occurring with MI.

Actually, the term dual diagnosis is a misnomer as many people may have other co-occurring disorders, such as medical disorders, in addition to IDD/MI.

Nevertheless, the term dual diagnosis has gotten traction over the last couple of decades and is often identified with the IDD/MI population.

Slide 4

This module covers basic information about the nature of Mental Health disorders among persons with Intellectual or Developmental Disabilities (IDD). The following content will be covered: definitions of IDD and mental illness, prevalence, indicators, common syndromes, characteristics, vulnerability factors, similarities and differences between MI and IDD.

Slide 5

Learning Objectives

- Define IDD
- Articulate prevalence rates
- Identify and describe 3 of the common syndromes
- Identify the four levels of severity
- Describe what is meant by "behavioral phenotype"
- Define MI
- Articulate prevalence rates
- Identify and describe DSM usage
- Define Dual Diagnosis
- Articulate prevalence rates
- Describe characteristics
- Describe vulnerability risk factors
- Articulate the similarities and differences between MI and IDD
- Describe four characteristics of persons with IDD/MI
- Describe vulnerability risk factors

Slide 6

> **Concept Of Dual Diagnosis**
>
> - **Co-Existence of Two Disabilities:**
>   **Intellectual/Developmental Disability (IDD) and**
>   **Mental Illness (MI)**
>
> - Both IDD and Mental Health disorders should
>   be assessed and diagnosed
> - **All needed treatments and supports should be**
>   **available, effective and accessible**

It is only within the past 35 years or so that professionals have recognized that it is possible for individuals to have both intellectual/developmental disability and mental illness.

Trained professionals are needed to conduct mental health assessment in people with IDD.

Services available for people with MI should also be available for people who have IDD/MI. Availability is not enough; we need staff who have a level of competency in dual diagnosis. The services need to be conducted by professionals who are trained in dual diagnosis. This helps to achieve effectiveness.

MODULE I

Slide 7

> ## Terminology
>
> The DSM 5 was published in May 2013 with many changes in diagnostic criteria and terminology.
>
> One of these is the change from the term "mental retardation" from DSM –IV to the term "intellectual disability" or "intellectual developmental disorder." This change better reflects terminology changes by medical, educational, service professionals and advocacy groups.
>
> DSM 5, 2013

Terminology in the DSM–5 is also reflective of new federal statute in the US – (Pub.L. 111-256, Rosa's Law). This law replaces the term "mental retardation" with "intellectual disability."

Intellectual developmental disorder is a disorder with onset during the developmental period that includes both intellectual and adaptive functioning deficits in conceptual, social, and practical domains. The three following criteria must be met:

- Deficits in intellectual functions, such as reasoning and problem solving, planning, abstract thinking, judgement, academic learning, and learning from experience, confirmed by both clinical assessment and individualized, standardized intelligence testing.

- Deficits in adaptive functioning that result in failure to meet developmental and sociocultural standards for personal independence and social responsibility. Without on-going support, the adaptive deficits limit functioning in one or more activities of daily life, such as communication, social participation, and independent living, across multiple environments, such as home, school, work, and community.

- Onset of intellectual and adaptive deficits during the developmental period. (American Psychiatric Association, 2013)

Together, these revisions bring DSM into alignment with terminology used by the World Health Organization's International Classification of Diseases, other professional disciplines and organizations, such as the American Association on Intellectual and Developmental Disabilities, and the U.S. Department of Education. (American Psychiatric Association, 2013)

Slide 8

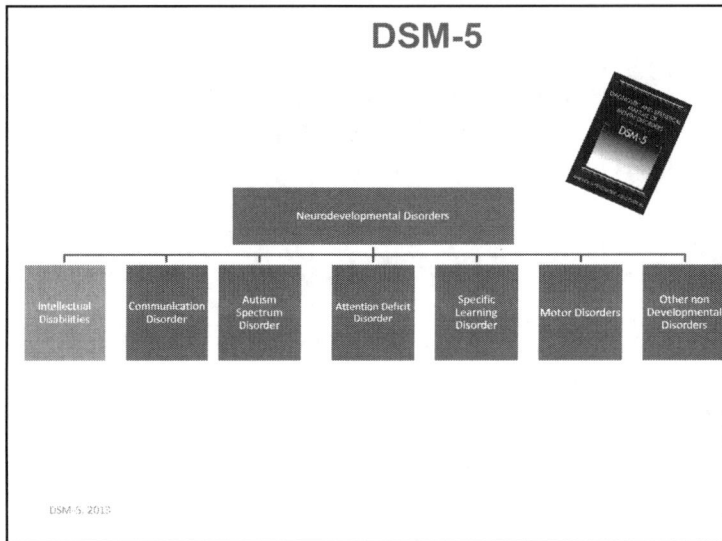

Neurodevelopmental disorders are deficiencies in growth and development of the brain or central nervous system. Included within the category of Neurodevelopmental Disorders in the DSM 5 is Intellectual Disability.

The DSM 5 includes in Neurodevelopmental Disorders:
- Intellectual Disability (Intellectual Developmental Disorder)
- Communication Disorder
- Attention Deficit Disorder
- Autism spectrum Disorder
- Specific Learning Disorder
- Motor Disorders
- Other non Developmental Disorders

Slide 9

Intellectual Developmental Disability – Diagnostic Criteria

Intellectual/Developmental Disorder

Following 3 diagnostic criteria must be met:

A. Deficits in intellectual functioning such as reasoning, problem solving, planning. Abstract thinking, academic learning and learning from experience, confirmed by both clinical assessment and individualized standardized testing;

B. Deficits in adaptive functioning that result in failure to meet developmental and sociocultural standards for personal independence and social responsibility. Without ongoing support, the adaptive deficits limit functioning in one or more activities of daily life, such as communication, social participation and independent living, across multiple environments such as home, school, work, and community.

C. Onset of intellectual and adaptive deficits during the developmental period.

DSM 5, 201

The criteria are based on adaptive functioning and not IQ scores because adaptive functioning determines the level of supports required. IQ scores alone do not give much information about the supports needed. Those are generally based on adaptive function and patterns of behavior.

Slide 10

Intellectual Developmental Disability – Three Domains

Disorder Characteristics: Three Domains

Intellectual/Developmental Disorder involves impairments of general mental abilities that impact adaptive functioning in three domains, or areas. These domains determine how well an individual copes with everyday tasks:

- The Conceptual Domain includes skills in language, reading, writing, math, reasoning, knowledge and memory.

- The Social Domain refers to empathy, social judgment, interpersonal communication skills, the ability to make and maintain friendships, and similar capacities

- The Practical Domain centers on self-management in areas such as personal care, job responsibilities, money management, recreation, and organizing school and work tasks.

DSM 5, 201

MODULE I

Adaptive functioning refers to a person's capacity to gain personal independence, based on the person's ability to learn and apply conceptual, social, and practical skills in his or her everyday life. As noted in the slide, adaptive functioning abilities are determined on the basis of the three domains: conceptual, social, and practical. Formal assessment will examine the level of functioning in each of the three domains.

Slide 11

Deficits in Adaptive Functioning

- **Self-care**

- **Language and communication**

- **Community use**

- **Independent living skills**

DM-ID, 2007

Deficits in adaptive behavior is one of the criteria to meet the definition of IDD. Deficits in adaptive behavior are also one of the three criteria to be eligible for services in the IDD system.

While change in terminology is reflected in federal statute, the federal Developmental Disabilities Act, 2000 (P.L. 106–402) still uses the term "developmental disability" and has not been formally updated.

Federal Definition of Developmental Disabilities
According to the Developmental Disabilities Act, section 102(8), "the term 'developmental disability' means a severe, chronic disability of an individual 5 years of age or older that:
- Is attributable to a mental or physical impairment or combination of mental and physical impairments;
- Is manifested before the individual attains age 22;

- Is likely to continue indefinitely;
- Results in substantial functional limitations in three or more of the following areas of major life activity;
    - (i) Self-care;
    - (ii) Receptive and expressive language;
    - (iii) Learning;
    - (iv) Mobility;
    - (v) Self-direction;
    - (vi) Capacity for independent living; and
    - (vii) Economic self-sufficiency.
- Reflects the individual's need for a combination and sequence of special, interdisciplinary, or generic services, supports, or other assistance that is of lifelong or extended duration and is individually planned and coordinated, except that such term, when applied to infants and young children means individuals from birth to age 5, inclusive, who have substantial developmental delay or specific congenital or acquired conditions with a high probability of resulting in developmental disabilities if services are not provided."

Slide 12

Deficits in Adaptive Functioning
(continued)

- Socialization skills
- Work
- Health and safety
- Self-direction

There is a clear trend for agencies to require identifiable and substantial deficits in adaptive behavior as one of the three criteria to meet eligibility for services. Assessment of functioning must consider typical behavior as opposed to optimal behavior.

There are several methods of adaptive function assessments including traditional, norm-referenced rating scales, and alternative methods. Considerations of best practice guidelines and benefits and limitations of each method should be considered before choosing the most appropriate/effective method for the particular assessment need.

Two of the more frequently used assessments for adaptive behavior are:
- The Vineland Adaptive Behavior Scales, Second Edition (Vineland-II) by Sara S. Sparrow, Domenic V. Cicchetti & David A. Balla, 2005. This measures adaptive behavior from birth to adulthood.
- The Adaptive Behavior Assessment System, second edition (ABAS-II; Harrison & Oakland, 2000), which uses a behavior-rating format to assess adaptive behavior and related skills for individuals 5 through 89 years of age.

Slide 13

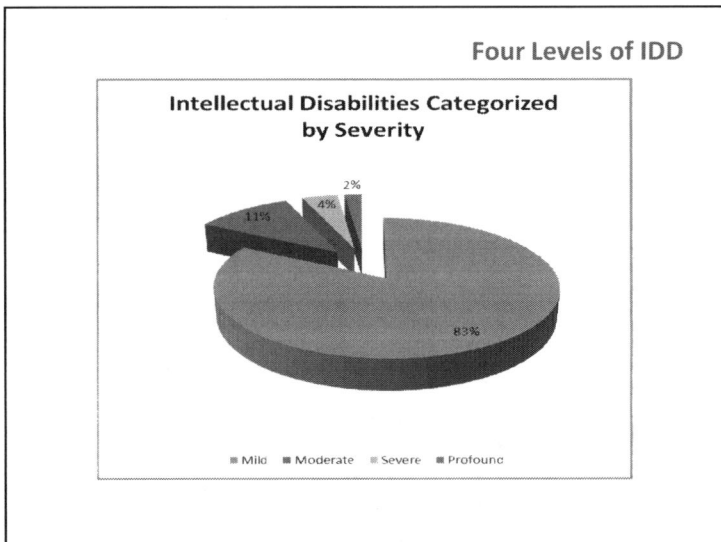

As 80-85% of people with IDD fall in the mild range, it is likely that the people you will come in contact with will have a certain degree of expressive and receptive language skills. The way in which we interact with persons in the mild range is not significantly different than the way we would interact with someone who does not have IDD.

Individuals with Mild IDD can often acquire academic skills and can become fairly self sufficient. Individuals with Moderate IDD can carry out work and self-care tasks with moderate supervision and are able to live and function successfully within the community, typically in a supervised environment. Individuals with Severe IDD may master very basic self-care skills and some communication skills. Individuals with Profound IDD may be able to develop limited self-care skills and some may learn to use communication devises with appropriate support and training. They generally need a high level of structure and supervision.

Slide 14

Four Levels of IDD

Mild: 80 – 85% of people with IDD
- Slower than normal development in all areas
- Unusual physiology rare
- Typical skill repertoire includes
  - practical skills
  - literacy skills
  - tasks of daily living/self-care
  - social skills

DSM5 2013

Note that as the person experiences greater levels of IDD, skill deficits become more significant, so instruction and supports become of paramount importance. Also as severity of IDD increases, the need for more precise/systematic means of instruction grows.

Slide 15

Four Levels of IDD

Moderate: 10 – 12 % of people with IDD

- **Noticeable delays, particularly speech**
- **May have unusual physiology**
- **Typical skills repertoire includes**
    - simple communication skills
    - simple health and safety skills
    - some tasks of daily living/self-care
    - independence in the community in familiar places

DSM 5, 2013

Slide 16

Four Levels of IDD

Severe: 3-4% of people with IDD

- **Significant delays in some areas**
- **May walk late**
- **Limited expressive communication skills**
- **Typical skills repertoire includes**
    - daily routines and repetitive activities
    - less complex tasks of daily living/self-care
    - social skills with support and supervision

DSM 5, 2013

Slide 17

Four Levels of IDD

Profound: 1-2% of people with IDD

- Significant delays in all areas
- Congenital abnormalities present
- Need close supervision
- Require specialized/attendant care
- May respond to regular physical and social activity
- Need intensive support to do self-care and activities of daily living

DSM 5, 2013

Slide 18

Exercise and Discussion

- What do you know about each of the severity levels of IDD (mild, moderate, severe, profound)?

- What is your personal experience with someone who has a disability?

Slide 19

Intellectual/Developmental
Disability - Causes

Thousands of Causes

- Chromosomal abnormalities
- Environmental genetic abnormalities
- Infections
- Metabolic issues/disorders
- Nutritional deficiencies/abnormalities
- Toxicity
- Trauma (Prenatal and perinatal)
- Unknown

Infections (present at birth or occurring after birth)
    Congenital CMV, Congenital rubella, Congenital toxoplasmosis
    Encephalitis, HIV infection, Listeriosis, Meningitis
Chromosomal abnormalities
    Chromosome deletions (such as cri du chat syndrome)
    Chromosomal translocations (a gene is located in an unusual spot on a
    chromosome, or located on a different chromosome than usual)
    Defects in the chromosome or chromosomal inheritance (such as frag-
    ile X syndrome, Angelman syndrome, Prader-Willi syndrome),
    Errors of chromosome numbers (such as Down syndrome)
Environmental
    Deprivation syndrome
Genetic abnormalities and inherited metabolic disorders
    Adrenoleukodystrophy, Galactosemia, Hunter syndrome, Hurler
    syndrome, Lesch-Nyhan syndrome, Phenylketonuria, Rett syndrome,
    Sanfilippo syndrome, Tay-Sachs disease, Tuberous sclerosis
Metabolic
    Congenital hypothyroid, Hypoglycemia (poorly regulated diabetes)
    Reye syndrome, Hyperbilirubinemia (very high bilirubin levels in babies)
Nutritional --Malnutrition
Toxic Intrauterine exposure to alcohol, cocaine, amphetamines, and other
drugs
    Lead poisoning, Methylmercury poisoning

Trauma (before and after birth)
> Intracranial hemorrhage before or after birth,
> Lack of oxygen to the brain before, during, or after birth
> Severe head injury

Unexplained (this largest category is for unexplained occurrences of intellectual disability)

Slide 20

```
                Common Types of Intellectual Developmental Disability


    • Down syndrome

    • Fragile X

    • Autism Spectrum Disorders (ASD)

    • Fetal Alcohol Spectrum Disorder (FASD)



  DM-ID, 2007
```

The most common syndromes associated with intellectual disabilities are Autism Spectrum Disorder, Down syndrome, Fragile X syndrome and Fetal Alcohol Spectrum Disorder (FASD).

MODULE I

Slide 21

Down Syndrome

Down syndrome is a genetic condition causing a set of delays in physical and intellectual development as a result of having an extra copy of chromosome 21.

National Down Syndrome Society (NDSS, 2012)

Down syndrome is a non-hereditary genetic mutation caused by an error in cell division which occurs at conception. It causes lifelong developmental delay and health complications of varying severity. According to the NIH, Down syndrome occurs in about 1 out of every 1,000 to 1,100 live births worldwide. (NDSS, 2012).

Slide 22

Down Syndrome

All people with Down syndrome experience cognitive delays, but the effect is usually mild to moderate.

NDSS, 2012

Slide 23

> **Down Syndrome**
>
> People who have Down syndrome have increased risk for
> certain medical conditions such as:
> - congenital heart defects
> - respiratory and hearing problems
> - Alzheimer's disease
> - childhood leukemia
> - thyroid conditions
>
> A few of the common physical traits of Down syndrome
> are low muscle tone, small stature, an upward slant to the
> eyes, and a single deep crease across the center of the
> palm.
>
> NDSS, 2013

Early interventions in specialized health care, speech therapy, physical therapy, and occupational therapy will improve outcomes for people who have Down syndrome.

Slide 24

> **Fragile X**
> - Fragile X syndrome is a genetic condition that
>   causes a range of developmental problems
>   including learning disabilities and cognitive
>   impairment.
>
> - Usually, males are more severely affected by this
>   disorder than females.
>
> - Fragile X syndrome does not always cause
>   intellectual disability, but most people who have
>   Fragile X have a mild or moderate intellectual
>   disability.
>
> DM-ID, 2007

M
O
D
U
L
E

I

Fragile X usually causes a mild to moderate intellectual disability, predisposition to anxiety and hyperactive behavior. About 1/3 of people who have Fragile X also have features of an autism spectrum disorder such as impairments with communication and social interactions.

As of 2013, there is a great deal of on-going research into the use of drug therapies to address the cellular and behavioral abnormalities of Fragile X.

Current therapies address the needs of a person who has Fragile X: speech and language, behavior, cognitive development, sensory integration. Medication is also often used to address some of the symptoms of Fragile X.

Slide 25

> **Autism Spectrum Disorder**
>
> **Autism Spectrum Disorder (ASD) is a complex condition that impacts normal brain development and affects a person's social relationships, communication, interests and behavior across multiple contexts. ASD is a single condition with different levels of symptom severity.**
>
> DSM 201

According to the DSM 5, ASD diagnosis now encompasses the previous DSM-IV autistic disorder, Asperger's Syndrome, childhood disintegrative disorder, and pervasive developmental disorder - not otherwise specified (PDD-NOS).

Under the DSM 5 diagnostic criteria, people with ASD must show symptoms from early childhood. This change in criteria encourages earlier diagnosis. People who have an ASD require different support levels depending of the severity of symptoms. Severity is based on social communication impairments and restricted, repetitive patterns of behavior (American Psychiatric Association, 2013).

There is ongoing research into to causes of ASD with a growing body of evidence for genetic causes in some cases.

Slide 26

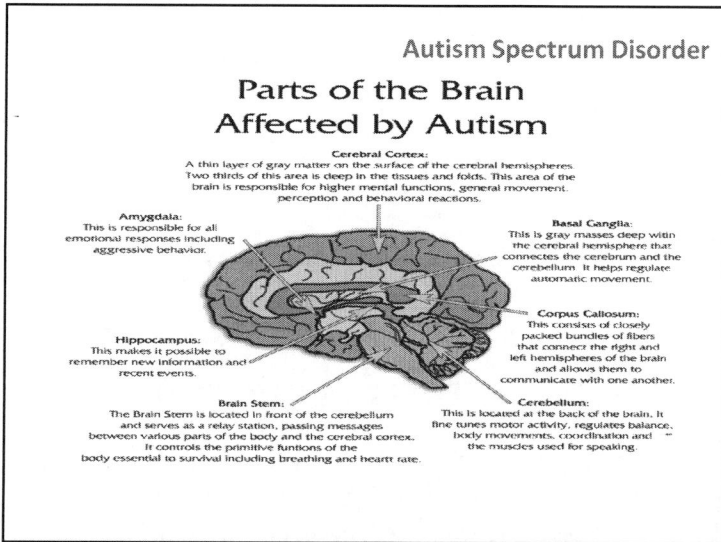

Magnetic resonance spectroscopy (MRS) can be used to detect regional concentrations of neuron-related molecules, a combination of altered molecular markers and an increase in white and gray matter (DiCicco-Bloom et al., 2006).

The core symptom domains likely involve widely dispersed neural systems and can imply generalized cellular abnormality. However, the differences in symptom severity and abilities can also suggest that not all brain systems are equally affected (DiCicco-Bloom et al., 2006).

Slide 27

> Autism Spectrum Disorder
>
> **ASD is characterized by:**
>
> - **Persistent deficits in social communication and social interaction across multiple contexts**
>
> **And**
>
> - **Restricted, repetitive patterns of behavior, interests, or activities**
>
> DSM 5, 201-

Diagnosis of ASD is based on the presence of both deficits in social communication and social interaction as well as restricted repetitive behaviors, interests, and activities. Symptoms must be present in the early developmental period; cause clinically significant impairment in social, occupational, or other important areas of current functioning; and are not better explained by intellectual disability or global developmental delay (American Psychiatric Association, 2013).

The diagnosis of ASD can now be made in children as young as 2 years as well as adults using a combination of standardized instruments: a parent interview (e.g., the Autism Diagnostic Interview–Revised) and an observational scale (e.g., the Autism Diagnostic Observation Schedule) (DiCicco-Bloom et al., 2006).

Diagnostic evaluation typically will involve a multi-disciplinary team: doctors (pediatrician), psychologist, speech and language pathologist, and occupational therapist. Genetic testing may likewise be recommended, as well as screening for related medical issues such as sleep difficulties.

Slide 28

> **Autism Spectrum Disorder**
>
> **People who have an autism spectrum disorder often have difficulties with:**
>
> - Social relationships
> - Transitions
> - Communication / language
> - Perseveration on interests and activities
> - Dependence on routine
> - Abnormal responses to sensory stimulation
>
> - Behavior problems
> - Variability of intellectual functioning
> - Uneven development profile
> - Difficulties in sleeping, toileting and eating
> - Immune irregularities
> - Nutritional deficiencies
> - Gastrointestinal problems
>
> DM-IC, 2003

Treatment of ASD usually focuses around early intervention with proper medical care, education/behavior therapy, language and speech therapy, occupational therapy, and physical therapy. The most significant impairments associated with an ASD are deficits in social relationships/interactions, deficits in communication, and variability of intellectual functioning.

Slide 29

> **Autism Spectrum Disorder**
>
> **ASD is typically noticed in the first or second year of life with:**
>
> - **delay or abnormality in language and play,**
> - **repetitive behaviors, such as spinning things or lining up small objects,**
> - **or unusual interests such as preoccupations with stop signs or ceiling fans.**
>
> DiCicco-Bloom, et al., 2006

Slide 30

> Autism Spectrum Disorder
>
> ### Common Strengths
>
> * Non-verbal reasoning skills
> * Reading skills
> * Perceptual motor skills
> * Drawing skills
> * Computer interest and skills
> * Exceptional memory
> * Visual spatial abilities
> * Music skills
>
> DSM-IV-TR, 2000

Although some areas of development in a person who has autism are delayed, people who have an autism spectrum disorder (ASD) often exhibit skills in other areas. These intellectual strengths may overshadow the developmental problems experienced.

Slide 31

> Autism Spectrum Disorder
>
> **Deficits in social communication can be observed in these areas:**
>
> * Delay in development of spoken language (no speech)
> * Lack of responses to the communications of others
> * Pronoun confusion (e.g., I vs. You)
> * Stereotypical and repetitive use of language (e.g., using lines from a favorite movie to communicate)
> * Idiosyncratic use of words and phrases (e.g., always salutes and says "Yes sir" when given a direction)
> * Abnormalities in pitch, stress, rate, rhythm, and intonation of speech
>
> McEvoy, Rogers, and Pennington, 2000

Deficits in communication/language – difficulties using and understanding verbal and non-verbal language are exceedingly common in people who have autism.

Slide 32

> **Autism Spectrum Disorder**
>
> **Deficits in social interaction can be observed in these areas:**
>
> - Failure to initiate or sustain conversations (e.g., turn taking)
> - Serious deficits in the ability to make friendships
> - Failure to respond to their names when called
> - Appearing not to listen when spoken to
> - Difficulty identifying boundaries of others
>
> McEvoy, Rogers, and Pennington, 2006

Autism is characterized by an impaired ability to engage in social relationships.

Slide 33

> **Autism Spectrum Disorder**
>
> **Restricted repetitive behaviors, interests and activities may be observed as:**
>
> - **Perseveration of interests and activities – people who have ASD typically have a narrow range of interests**
> - **Repetitive, stereotyped body movements such as hand flicking, spinning or rocking**
> - **Perseverations might extend to food**
> - **Dependence on routine**
>
> McEvoy, Rogers, and Pennington, 2006

Difficulties in sleeping, toileting, and eating are common in people who have an ASD.

Abnormal responses to sensory stimulation are also common. Many people who have ASDs have unexpected reactions to stimuli. People may have hyper-sensitivity (cannot tolerate touch, can hear the sound of a light buzzing, can be fascinated with an object spinning, etc.) or hyposensitivity (can appear deaf, extremely high pain tolerance to different sensory stimuli).

Slide 34

Fetal Alcohol Spectrum Disorder
(FASD)

FASD is a term used to describe a range of disabilities caused by pre-natal exposure to alcohol.

Astley & Clarren, 2002

Diagnosis is based on a history of prenatal alcohol consumption by the mother, combined with a group of characteristics in the infant: poor growth, character-istic facial features, and neurological abnormalities.

Slide 35

> FASD
>
> The 4-digit Diagnostic Code provides a reproducible, objective, consistent and precise method for the diagnosis of FAS. Four criteria are assessed, quantified and assigned a rating of 1 to 4 for each criteria, depending on the degree of abnormality:
>
> * impaired growth;
> * facial abnormalities;
> * abnormal brain function; and
> * degree of maternal drinking.
>
> Astley & Claren, 1999

Pre-natal exposure to alcohol causes IDD in approximately 10% of all cases. However, it is still one of the leading causes of preventable intellectual disability (Astley & Claren, 1999).

Slide 36

> FASD
>
> **While each person impacted by FASD is unique, brain damage typically results in various dysfunctional behavioral symptoms commonly found with this disability.**
>
> Astley & Claren, 2000

MODULE I

Dysfunctional behavior symptoms include:
- Memory problems
- Difficulty storing and retrieving information
- Inconsistent performance ("on" and "off") days
- Impulsivity, distractibility, disorganization
- Ability to repeat instructions, but inability to put them into action ("talk the talk but don't walk the walk")
- Difficulty with abstractions, such as math, money management, time concepts
- Cognitive processing deficits (may think more slowly)
- Slow auditory pace (may only understand every third word of normally paced conversation)
- Developmental lags (may act younger than chronological age)
- Inability to predict outcomes or understand consequence

(Streissguth, Barr, Kogan, & Bookstein, 1996; Steissguth & Kanter, 1997)

Slide 37

Secondary characteristics can be prevented with proper diagnosis and support strategies.

Intervention strategies typically include concrete instructions, consistent messages, repetition, routine, simple tasks, explanations, supervision, and decreased stimulation (Streissguth, et. al., 1996).

Slide 38

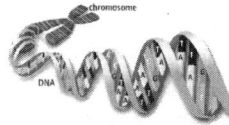

The genome is an organism's complete set of DNA. Genomes vary widely in size: the smallest known genome for a free-living organism (a bacterium) contains about 600,000 DNA base pairs, while human and mouse genomes have some 3 billion. Except for mature red blood cells, all human cells contain a complete genome.

DNA in the human genome is arranged into 24 distinct chromosomes--physically separate molecules that range in length from about 50 million to 250 million base pairs. A few types of major chromosomal abnormalities, including missing or extra copies or gross breaks and rejoinings (translocations), can be detected by microscopic examination. Most changes in DNA, however, are more subtle and require a closer analysis of the DNA molecule to find perhaps single-base differences.

Slide 39

Phenotype and Genotypes

Definition of Phenotype:

The phenotype of a genetic syndrome is the set of physical characteristics produced by a genetic abnormality or genotype (DM-ID, 2009).

Definition of Behavioral Phenotype:

The specific and characteristic repertoire exhibited by people with a genetic disorder (Flint & Yule, 1994).

It is important to recognize the roles that behavioral phenotypes play. If we fail to pay attention to them, we can miss an important means for understanding the nature of challenges that some people present. Not all people, but some.

Slide 40

Fragile X Phenotype

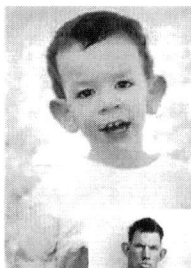

Long face, prominent ears, high arched palate, flat feet, soft skin, other connected tissue abnormalities (DM-ID 2007)

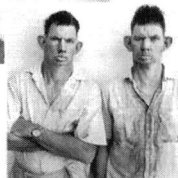

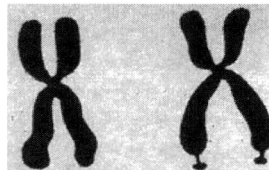

Anxiety—hyperarousal
Early signs—self injury(hand wrist biting), mouthing objects, hand flapping
Escalate to task refusal, leaving the area, verbal aggression with imitated phrases
Triggers—forced eye contact, personal space issues, tactile defensiveness, emotional tone of peers/staff, changes in routine, auditory stimuli
Other contributors—auditory processing deficits, delayed emotional processing, hypersensitivity to negative correction, poor concept of time

A "cure" for Fragile X which targets pharmaceutical treatments is undergoing human clinical trials. It will target the underlying biochemical pathway affected by the Fragile X gene mutation.
Families diagnosed with Fragile X syndrome will be able to benefit from this medical breakthrough.

Slide 41

Behavioral Phenotypes in Youth with Fragile X Syndrome

Social anxiety, shyness, gaze aversion, perseveration, autism/PDD, inattention, hyperactivity, sadness or depression (primarily females), Attention Deficit Disorder

X-linked (carriers: F-1:259; M-1:800)
1:2000 males; 1:4000 females
FMR1 gene on X chromosome (Xq27.3)
        Normal 0 to 25 repeats
        Premutation-25 to 200 repeats
        Mutation >200 repeats
Diagnosis: DNA testing for mutation via PCR

FRAGILE X SYNDROME
Facial features:
      Long face
      Large, protuberant ears
Hyperextensible joints especially fingers
Flat feet
Large size
Macroorchidism
Cognition:
      Males most with IDD
      Females 1/3 to ½ with IDD, others with Learning Disability (LD)
ADHD (M-80-90%)
Anxiety Disorders
Mood disorders e.g. bipolar disorder/depression
Autism (15-33%)/Autistic characteristics
      Handflapping/Pica
      Poor social judgment/interaction
      Sound/light/texture sensitivity
      Poor eye contact/perseverative speech

Slide 42

Phenotype:
Williams Syndrome

Full lips, puffy cheeks, small jaw, short statue, spinal curvature, slumped posture (DM-ID, 2007)

Slide 43

> **Behavioral Phenotypes in Youth with Williams Syndrome**
>
> **Anxiety, fears, phobias, inattention, hyperactivity, social disinhibiting, overly friendly, indiscriminate relating, Attention Deficit Disorder**

Highly characteristic facial abnormalities, cardiac abnormalities, metabolic problems - high blood calcium levels
Contiguous gene sequence, Deletion chromosome 7
1:20,000 births general pop, 1 in 100 with IDD
Associated IDD, mild to moderate IDD

Appealing face & engaging smile, auditory processing strength; strength in musical ability and facial recognition
Short attention span/ADHD
Cocktail party chatter—well developed verbal skills, no fear of strangers
Obsessive compulsive characteristics e.g. topic of conversation
Unusually sensitive to noise (hyperacusis), fear of heights
Difficulty building friendships, poor visual motor integration, medically fragile
Nail-biting, skin picking behaviors
Anxiety/anxiety disorders
Autism/autistic features

Slide 44

Prader-Willi Phenotype

Hyperphagia, obesity, small hands and feet, dysmorphic facial features (DM-ID, 2007)

Victor at 1 year
Behavioral problems--low frustration tolerance, socialization difficulties, temper tantrums, OC tendencies, rituals, impulsivity, skin picking

Weight control—obesity can be prevented 1000 to 1200 calorie diet with 30 minutes exercise—locking up food—consider growth hormone since many have GH deficiency (as of 2000, GH became a treatment for PWS)—slightly controversial

Slide 45

Behavioral Phenotypes in Youth
with Prader-Willi

- **Hyperphagia, non-food obsessions & compulsions, skin-picking, temper tantrums, perseveration, stubbornness, under activity, OCD, Affective Disorders**

General population 1 in 15,000 with IDD, 1 in 100

Hypotonia in utero (decreased fetal movement) infancy with Failure to Thrive in first year of life; weak cry, delayed motor milestones —delayed walking until 2 years
Short stature
Hypogonadism
Hyperphagia—food seeking behavior, hoarding, eating inedible materials, leading to morbid obesity
Low muscle tone leads to exercise aversion
Average IQ around 70-good expressive language
Skin picking
Variable cognition—strength in visual processing
Low tolerance for teasing, try to hide overeating, nurturing tends to get "stuck on topics"

Slide 46

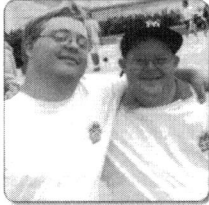

Down Syndrome Phenotype

Small head, upward slant eyes, broad neck, hearing loss, obesity, gastrointestinal problems (DM-ID, 2007)

TRISOMY 21-Down syndrome
Major malformations
      Cardiac
      GI
Minor malformations
      Facial, skin, etc
Developmental pattern
      IDD
      Learning pattern

Slide 47

Behavioral Phenotypes in Youth with Down Syndrome

Noncompliance, stubbornness, inattention, over activity, argumentative, withdrawn (depression and dementia among adults), ADHD

ADHD
Autism
      In about 8% of people
      (Kent, Evans, Paul, & Sharp, 1999)
Alzheimer Dementia
      16-50% depending on criteria for diagnosis
      May require different programs than typical for IDD

MODULE I

Slide 48

Behavioral Phenotypes

Behavioral phenotypes

- **Are not set in stone**
- **Look at syndromes rather than set diagnoses**
- **Behavioral manifestations arise from the interaction of genes and environment**
- **Present a wide range of symptoms**
- **Used as clues not as expectations**

Characterizing behavioral phenotype of a specific genetic disorder is a relatively recent approach to studying "mental retardation syndromes" (Accardo and Capute, 1998). It involves characterizing the behavioral phenotype of a specific genetic disorder (Finegan, 1998; O'Brien & Yule, 1995; Simonoff, Bolton, & Rutter, 1998).

Advances in behavioral phenotype research occur in two ways:

- Studying individuals with known genetic disorders such as Fragile X syndrome and developing syndrome characterizations based on the observation.
- Looking for a genetic marker in people with behavioral commonalities. For example, the behavioral phenotype and developmental course of Rett syndrome has been well documented (Hagberg and Witt-Engerstrom, 1986) but until recently, the genetic marker had not been identified. As Rett syndrome previously has an identifiable phenotype without a genetic marker it remained in the DSM IV as an acceptable psychiatric diagnosis. Since the discovery of the genetic marker, it does not appear as a psychiatric diagnosis in the DSM – 5. This has been the case with other genetically based syndromes such as Down syndrome or Fragile X syndrome, which are not included.

Etiologically based diagnosis is beneficial in driving clinical treatment and the related individual supports for a person. It is much easier to develop a unified support system when professionals, the family, and the individual are operating from a common unifying concept such as an etiological diagnosis.

Slide 49

> ### Mental Health Problems vs. Mental Illness
>
> People occasionally experience mental health problems that may:
>
> - Change the way they think and understand the world around them
>
> - Change the way they interrelate with others
>
> - Change the emotions and feelings they have
>
> These changes can have a short-term impact on the way they deal with day-to-day life.
>
> However, if the impact is very great (ongoing problems with repeated relapse episodes) then we consider the possibility of mental illness.

From time to time, we all experience situations in our lives that contribute to increased stress and anxiety. These are usually externally driven. That is to say, impacts from environmental/social situations can cause a great deal of stress in our lives. These stressors can contribute to short-term anxiety and worry. For example, moving from one home to another can be an extremely stressful situation but that stress will only last for a limited time.

However, when the impact of the stressful situation continues for a long period of time, i.e., over 3 months, and the severity of the stress interferes with day-to-day functioning, then we are looking at more than just a mental health problem. If the stressful situation goes on for a period of time and has frequent and intense episodes, then we may be looking at mental illness rather than just a mental health problem.

MODULE I

Slide 50

> **What Is Mental Illness (MI)?**
>
> • MI is a psychiatric condition that disrupts a person's thinking, feeling, mood, ability to relate to others, and can impair daily functioning.
>
> • MI can affect persons of any age, race, religion, income, or level of intelligence.
>
> • The DSM 5 or the DM-ID provide diagnostic criteria for mental disorders.
>
> DSM 5, 201*

"A mental disorder (mental illness) is a syndrome characterized by clinically significant disturbance in an individual's cognition, emotion regulation, or behavior that reflects dysfunction in the psychological, biological, or developmental processes underlying mental functioning. Mental disorders are usually associated with significant distress or disability in social, occupational, or other important activities" (American Psychiatric Association, 2013).

A mental illness is a psychological or behavioral pattern generally associated with subjective stress. A mental illness may consist of a combination of affective, behavioral, cognitive, and perceptual components.

Onset of mental illness generally occurs at late adolescence or early adulthood. However, all ages are susceptible.

Slide 51

What Is Mental Illness? (cont.)

Mental illness is a biological process that affects the brain. Some refer to it as a brain disorder.

DSM 5, 2013

Emerging science indicates that most psychiatric disorders are biologically driven. We are finding that brain abnormalities are the cause of many serious mental illnesses.

Mental disorders can arise from a combination of sources. In many cases, there is no single accepted or consistent cause currently established.

For people who have ID, current thinking is that there is likely to be bio-psycho-social influences that contribute to the development of mental illness in persons with ID.

MODULE I

Slide 52

> Vulnerabilities
>
> Mental illnesses (mental disorders) can also be defined as a variety of psychiatric conditions which may be a result of vulnerabilities in:
>
> * Environment
> * Biology
> * Psychosocial factors
>
> DSM 3, 2013

Environmental factors can include:
* poverty
* interrupted nurturing in adolescence/childhood
* substance abuse
* work/school problems
* abuse
* rejection by others
* stressful relationships
* low social supports
* major life events

Psychosocial factors can create vulnerability due to a number of differing conditions that have a high influence on mental illness: poor social skills, poor coping skills, communication problems, etc.

Family history of mental illness creates strong vulnerability for a person experiencing mental illness or symptoms themselves. Studies suggest this influence relates primarily to genetics as opposed to early family environments. (Goldberg, 2001)

Biological factors that can increase vulnerability to mental illness include: family history of certain psychosis, brain abnormalities, neurodevelopmental problems, disease, prenatal nutrition and health, etc.

Slide 53

> Definition Of Mental Illness In Persons With Intellectual/Developmental Disability
>
> ## Criteria
>
> **1. When behavior is abnormal by virtue of quantitative or qualitative differences.**
>
> 2. When behavior cannot be explained on the basis of developmental delay alone.
>
> **3. When behavior causes significant impairment in functioning.**
>
> Adapted from Einfeld & Aman, 1995

This definition applies to individuals who have an intellectual disability.

Three criteria are required to identify mental illness in persons with IDD:

- Maladaptive behavior is observed and there is a difference, in frequency or content of the behavior, from baseline.
- The maladaptive behavior, which is a change from baseline, is not directly as result of the IDD.
- Maladaptive behavior, which is a change from baseline, results in impairment in day-to-day functioning over time (Einfeld & Aman, 1995).

Slide 54

> **A Summary Of Similarities And Differences**
> **Between Intellectual/Developmental Disability**
> **(IDD) & Mental Illness (MI)**
>
> **IDD:**   **refers to sub-average functional intellect**
> MI: has nothing to do with intellect
>
> **IDD:**   **incidence: 1-2% of general population**
> MI: incidence: 16-20% of general population
>
> **IDD:**   **present at birth or occurs before age 18**
> MI: may have its onset at any age (usually late adolescent)

There are many differences between IDD and MI. Nevertheless, a person with IDD can have MI.

It has only been in the past four decades that we have realized or understood that people with IDD can have co-occurring MI.

Slide 55

> A Summary Of Similarities And Differences
> Between Intellectual/Developmental
> Disability (IDD) & Mental Illness (MI)
>
> **IDD:** **functional intellectual impairment is permanent**
>
> MI: often temporary and may be reversible and is often cyclic
>
> **IDD:** **a person can usually be expected to behave rationally at his or her developmental level**
>
> MI: a person may vacillate between normal and irrational behavior, displaying degrees of each

It is important to realize the differences between chronological age and developmental age in a person who has IDD.

Behavior observed in people at the lower end of the IQ scale may, at first appearance, look like maladaptive behavior. For example, self talk and imaginary friends are typical behaviors observed in young children in the neurotypical population. Although self talk and imaginary friends in neurotypical adults may be indicative of a mental illness, it could be normal in persons who have ID. For example, an adult age 20 with an IQ of 45 may exhibit self talk or have an imaginary friend. This is because his developmental age can closely match the developmental age of a 4 year old child.

Slide 56

> # Exercise
>
> What did you learn from this section regarding people who have IDD/MI?

Slide 57

Comparison Between IDD and MI

Intellectual/Developmental Disability	Mental Illness
Below-average ability to learn and to use information	Inappropriate thought processes &/or emotions
Before adulthood	Can occur anytime in a person's life
Refers to sub-average functional intellect	Has nothing to do with intellect
Lifelong. There is no cure.	May be temporary, cyclic, or episodic. May be curable
Services involve training and education not medication	Services involve therapy and medication
Is not psychiatric in nature	Diagnosed illnesses such as Depression, Schizophrenia, Bi-Polar Disorder
Impairments in social skills and adaptations	Does not necessarily impact social competence
Behavior is usually rational	Behavior may vacillate between normal and irrational

Slide 58

Prevalence of MI in IDD

Two to four times

a typical population

(Corbett 1979)

40% of people with IDD have co-occurring MI

(Einfeld and Tongue, 1996)

44% of people with IDD have MI

(Nci, 20145)

Researchers have found that one third or more of people with IDD have significant behavioral, mental, or personality disorder requiring mental health services.

Research studies have had a varied range of mental illness in persons with IDD. This is because of differing research methods (assessment methodology, in-patient or out-patient populations, differing definitions, etc.). However, the research and professional community have recognized and accepted a prevalence rate of at least one third of individuals who have IDD would warrant having a co-occurring psychiatric disorder.

MODULE I

Slide 59

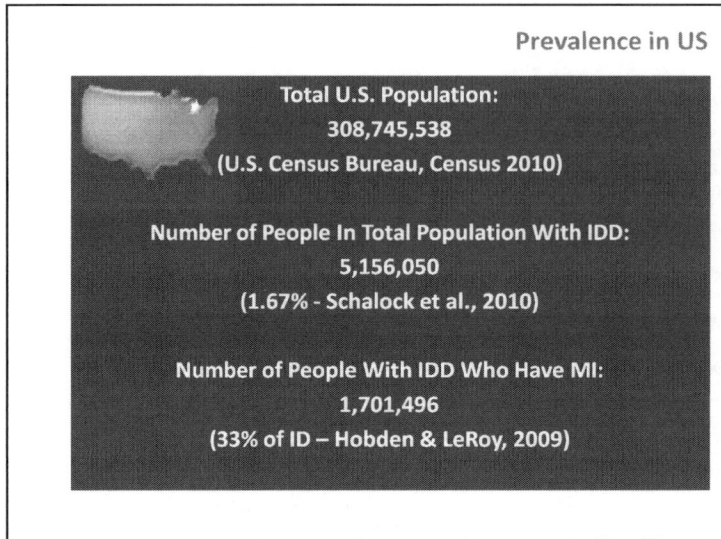

Recent census indicates there are over 300 million people in the United States.

Research indicates that approximately 1.6% of the general population have IDD, which accounts for more than 5 million people.

NADD has embraced the prevalence rate of one third of people with IDD having a co-occurring MI disorder, resulting in an estimate of somewhat over a million and a half people with a dual diagnosis in the U.S.

Slide 60

Prevalence Canada

Total Canada Population

35,141,542

(Government of Canada, Statistics Canada, 2015)

Number of People in Total Population with IDD:

586,864

(1.67% - Schalock et al., 2010)

Number of People With IDD Who Have MI:

193,665

(33% of ID – Hobden & LeRoy, 2009)

Slide 61

Indicators

Signs a person with IDD may have an MI

Increased anxiety, panic or fright	Excessive reactivity / moodiness
Hearing, seeing, feeling imaginary things (hearing voices is not the same as talking to oneself for company, to process thoughts, or self-talk to reduce anxiety)	Memory problems (worsening memory or change in memory)
Need for instant fulfillment / gratification	Accelerated speech patterns
Unusual sleep patterns (insomnia or lengthy periods of sleep)	Changes in appetite (loss of weight or increase in weight)
False beliefs (delusional thinking or paranoia)	Heightened emotional sensitivity

Slide 62

Signs a person with IDD may have an MI Continued

• Decline in personal hygiene	• Self-isolation
• Inappropriate expressive reactions	• Lingering sadness
• Family history of mental illness	• Self-injurious behavior
• A functional or behavioral change	• Suicidal ideation

Slide 63

Consider this person

Nguyen is a 48 year old man with Down syndrome. He recently has begun to refuse previously enjoyed activities and occasionally becomes agitated when prompted to get ready for work in the morning, preferring to stay in bed all day with the lights out. His family and in home staff are frustrated with him and one person has stated that he is just plain lazy. Could this be depression?

Slide 64

Recent research has indicated that people with IDD are more vulnerable to stress than people who do not have IDD. Situations that may not result in stress for a neurotypical person may cause a great deal of stress for a person with IDD.

For example, meeting new people and interacting is a normative behavior for the neurotypical person. However, for a person who has IDD, meeting new people and interacting with them may create a very stressful situation.

Vulnerability to stress can also be a product of limited life experience, limited opportunities and options, expectations that can exceed their abilities, and past learning experiences. People who have IDD can develop mental health problems when confronted with only minimal to moderate stress.

Slide 65

> ### Characteristics Of People With IDD/MI
>
> •Challenges with coping skills
>
> • Stress management difficulties
>
> • Fewer wellness opportunities
>
> • Frequently lack the basic skills required for everyday living; e.g., budgeting money, using public transportation, doing laundry, preparing meals, etc.

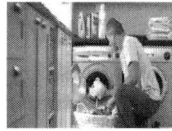

Individuals with IDD usually need instruction on how to perform basic responsibilities in daily life. This is particularly important for people living in the community. These tasks and functions need to be taught in a step-by-step manner with repetition as a method of learning. Instruction and teaching can be done either in the natural environment (home) or in a more formal environment (day program, school, work/employment).

Slide 66

Characteristics Of People With IDD/MI

Extreme Dependency

Often experience themselves as quite helpless, thus requiring massive support from families or care providers to live successfully

Hartline & McLean, 2004

Due to dependency on caregivers, mental health may suffer if that support is removed or threatened. Helping the person develop his/her independence and resiliency as much as possible can assist with addressing this vulnerability.

Slide 67

Characteristics of People with IDD/MI

Difficulty with Interpersonal Relationships

- **With some exceptions, people with IDD/MI often have great difficulty in developing and maintaining close relationships with others.**

- **These interpersonal relationship problems can result in disruption in school, home, work, and social environments.**

Hartline & McLean, 2004

MODULE I

People with IDD/MI can have disruptions, across the lifespan, because of challenges associated with interpersonal relationships. These challenges can interfere in several domains involved in the individual's life.

For children, the challenge of interpersonal relationships can result in parent-child conflicts. For school-aged children, this challenge can occur with school-aged peers as well as with teachers. For adults, the problems associated with interpersonal relationships can interfere with social relationships, as well as causing problems at work and problems at the residential environment.

People with a dual diagnosis, have difficulty in developing symmetrical relationships with others. These individuals often do not understand nor apply a "give and take" relationships with others. In part this is due to a history of authority figures interacting with the individual. The nature of the relationship is usually unequal, and this inequality of relationships carries through the lifespan.

Individuals need to be taught how to engage in interpersonal relationships that are appropriate to the context in which the interpersonal relationship occurs. Formal social skills learning is needed to assist these individuals in developing and maintaining interpersonal relationships.

Additionally, the co-occurring mental illness can interfere with ongoing and appropriate interpersonal relationships. For example, an individual who has a psychotic disorder and is not stable is likely to have challenges in appropriate interpersonal relationships. The symptoms associated with an active psychotic disorder can significantly interfere with how the individual interacts with others.

Slide 68

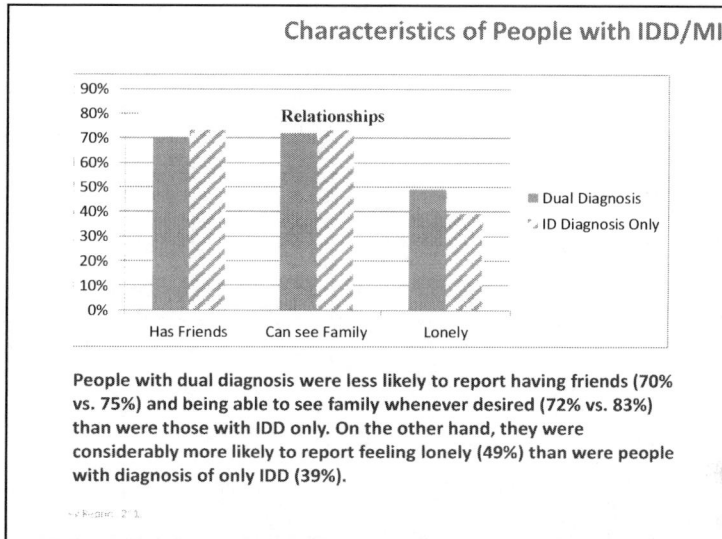

Characteristics of People with IDD/MI

Relationships

■ Dual Diagnosis
ID Diagnosis Only

Has Friends   Can see Family   Lonely

People with dual diagnosis were less likely to report having friends (70% vs. 75%) and being able to see family whenever desired (72% vs. 83%) than were those with IDD only. On the other hand, they were considerably more likely to report feeling lonely (49%) than were people with diagnosis of only IDD (39%).

Developing meaningful relationships is difficult for people with a dual diagnosis. Also, the feeling of loneliness occurs in nearly 50% of people with IDD/MI.

It is important to assist people in nurturing and developing relationships. This can be accomplished in a variety of environments including school, habilitative programs, as well as individual/group therapy.

Once individuals with a dual diagnosis begin to develop meaningful relationships, their feeling(s) of loneliness often subside.

MODULE I

Slide 69

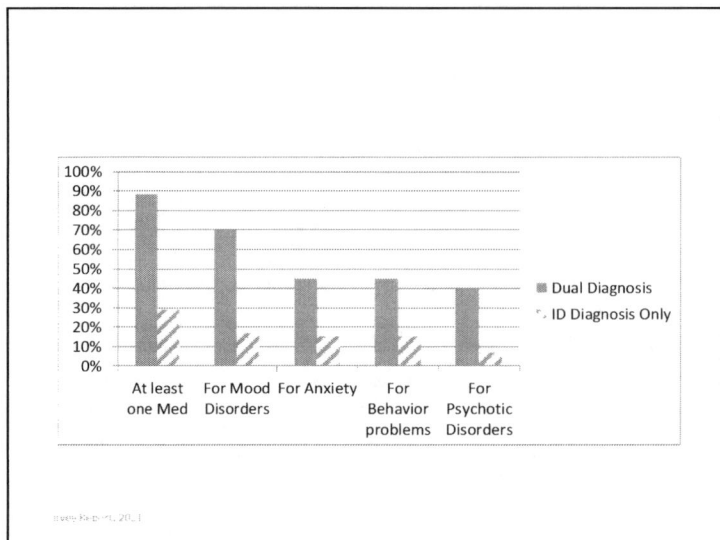

Not surprisingly, people with dual diagnosis were much more likely than people with only an IDD diagnosis to take at least one kind of psychotropic medication. The biggest difference was in the proportion of people taking medication for mood disorders – 70% of people with a dual diagnosis were taking them, compared to 17% with IDD diagnosis only.

What is more surprising is the finding that 29% of people without a diagnosis of mental illness take at least one type of psychotropic medication. This indicates that nearly one third of people with IDD are being prescribed psychotropic medications for behavioral control. In the US, there has been a history of prescribing these kinds of medications for people with IDD to suppress behavioral problems.

Psychotropic medication treatment should be used only after a mental illness has been diagnosed. Prescribing medication treatment can be effective, but should be used only when it is related to a specific psychiatric diagnosis.

Slide 70

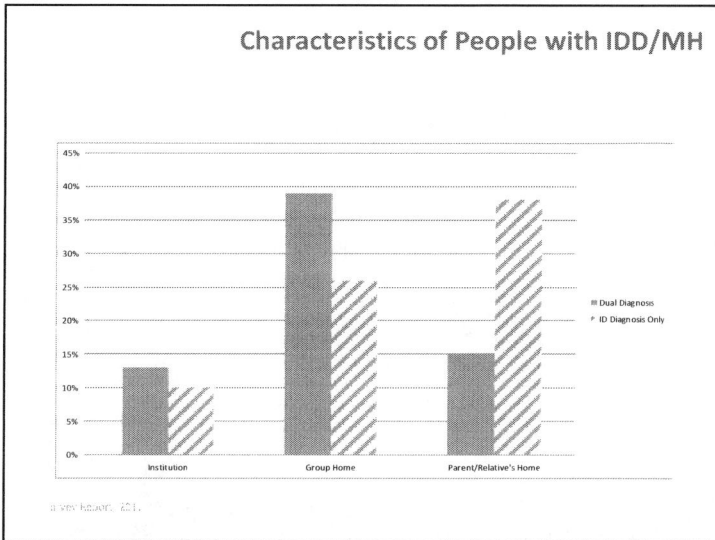

As a group, individuals with dual diagnosis were more likely to live in a group home, 39% compared to 26% for those with IDD only, and less likely to live in a parent/relative's home, 15% compared to 38%.

It is likely that behavioral/psychiatric problems are one contributor to why, as a group, individuals with a dual diagnosis are more likely to live in a group home than those who have IDD only. Similarly, this group of people are less likely to live with parents/relatives than people with IDD only. People with a dual diagnosis usually need a structured environment and a higher level of support with secondary issues such as medication and symptom management. Group home living environments may offer more structure than living in parents'/relatives' home environments.

MODULE I

Slide 71

Characteristics of People with IDD/MI

Difficulty Working in the Competitive Job Market

People with IDD/MI often have difficulty working in a competitive employment. They may have frequent job changes interspersed with long periods of unemployment.

Persons with IDD/MI often have difficulty in both obtaining and sustaining employment in the competitive market. Behavioral problems often interfere with their ability to maintain job performance.

The behavioral problems may be triggered by perceived stress within the work environment or outside the work environment. Alternatively, the work distribution could be caused by an exacerbation or decompensation related to their mental illness.

Job coaching may help a person with IDD/MI in a work environment. The job coach would be able to assess if the person is experiencing stress and can function as a liaison between the individual and the work environment.

Slide 72

	Characteristics of People with IDD/MH				
Employment (community job)					
	Hours worked in 2 weeks	Amount earned in two weeks	Hourly Wage	Earning at or above minimum wage (%)	Length at current job
Dual Diagnosis	30.6	$170	$5.81	35%	56 months
IDD Only	31.5	$201	$6.40	43%	66 months

NCI Survey Report, 2010

Slightly fewer people with a dual diagnosis reported having a job in the community than people with an IDD diagnosis only (22% vs. 27%).

People with only IDD earned $201 on average in the most recent typical two week time period preceding interview, whereas people with dual diagnosis earned $170 on average; the number of hours worked in the same time period was similar (31.5 and 30.6 respectively).

The data indicates that fewer people with a dual diagnosis are employed in the community compared to those with IDD only, and those with a dual diagnosis who are employed make less money than those who have IDD only.

MODULE I

Slide 73

Characteristics of People with IDD/MI

- People with IDD/MI may learn more slowly.
- They may have difficulty recalling information – especially newly required information.

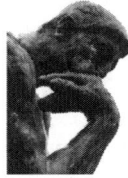

Memory issues and difficulty learning are quite common for people with IDD. Assisting them to learn to use memory tools and modifying learning/teaching requirements to level of ability improves the person's ability to be successful with these tasks.

Slide 74

Characteristics of People with IDD/MI

- May have difficulty focusing, may have shortened attention span
- Difficulty in understanding some abstract concepts
- May have difficulty in considering alternative solutions. For example, may see things in "black and white" terms.

Strategies to modify requirements about prolonged attention to task and decision making skills can greatly assist a person who has IDD in these areas. Using concrete language and avoiding the use of slang and jargon can make a great difference in the person's ability to grasp concepts and communication.

Slide 75

Characteristics of People with IDD/MI

- May have difficulty generalizing skills sets

- Developed skill sets may be very task specific

- Passive learning style which may make it difficult for the trainer to know what information is being retained

- Low expectations due to past difficulties. "Self fulfilled prophecy"- the individual believes he/she can not learn, thus preventing learning.

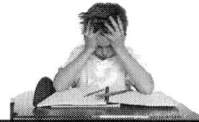

MODULE I

Slide 76

Characteristics of People with IDD/MI

Exercise

Can you share examples of what might assist a person with IDD through some of the learning issues on the previous slide?

Ask the participants to give examples of what might assist a person with IDD through these learning issues.
Examples could include:
Strategies to gain attention: using the person's name frequently
Positive support strategies
Errorless learning strategies (set the person up for success)

Slide 77

> **Characteristics of People with IDD/MI**
>
> - May "perseverate" on some things
>
> - Much harder to focus on things that are too difficult
>
> - Problems with cognitive rigidity:
>
>   - ❖ Difficulty changing from one task to another
>   - ❖ Difficulty accepting alternative solutions or explanations
>   - ❖ Difficulty shifting focus of attention

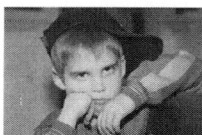

Transitions from a preferred activity to a less preferred activity can be very difficult for a person with IDD. Attention to how to set up transitions and shift focus can assist the person to move through his or her perseveration to a new task.

Slide 78

> **Characteristics of People with IDD/MI**
>
> - Being different from peers
> - Losses rather than gains
> - Social isolation although mainstreamed
> - Rejected by peers
> - Failure experiences dominate school histories
> - Low social status

M
O
D
U
L
E

I

Ask the participants to give examples of how a person with IDD might experience each of these points.

Some responses might be:
Being bullied and picked on or left out of activities
Being picked last for teams
Watching peers succeed academically much more quickly than they are

Slide 79

Characteristics of People with IDD/MI

- **Outer directed personality orientation**
  - look to others rather than selves for problem solution
- **Aberrant social styles:**
  - ❖**Too wary or too disinhibited**
  - ❖**Low expectancy or enjoyment of success**

Issues related to higher dependency on care givers, isolation from natural peer group and difficulty learning social skills create difficulty for a person with IDD when trying to fit in with a group or to make friends. Skills that are learned typically through observing and imitating the actions of others may need to be taught more directly using positive reinforcement, modelling, or verbal cueing in smaller steps.

Slide 80

Characteristics Of People With IDD/MI

- Low self-esteem
- Distrust of self
- Sadness, depression, dependency & withdrawal
- Helplessness
- Impulsivity

Fein & Bennett Gull, 1997

There is a large body of research showing that low self-esteem is a more significant issue for people who have an IDD than for their non-disabled peers.

Helping the person identify and focus on his or her strengths as well as building skills in other areas, can assist in building self-esteem. This can have a large impact on preventing mental health issues related to low self-esteem.

MODULE I

Slide 81

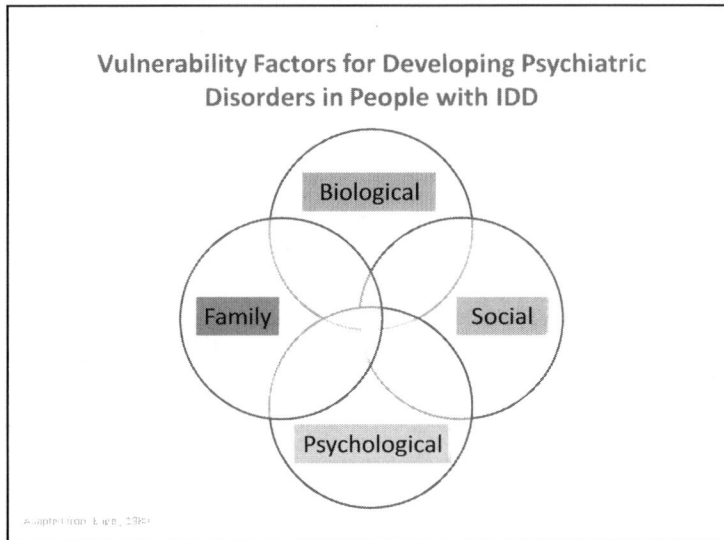

Vulnerability Factors for Developing Psychiatric Disorders in People with IDD

Biological

Family

Social

Psychological

Adapted from Lue, 390?

Very little is known about the causes of mental illness in people with IDD. However, it is proposed that there are both internal and external influences that contribute to the high rate of mental disorders in persons with IDD.

There are several risk factors that predispose people with IDD to develop psychiatric disorders. There are biological, psychological, and social circumstances that contribute vulnerability to mental health disorders in persons with IDD.

Slide 82

There are a number of circumstances causing or contributing to mental health disorders in person with IDD. People with IDD are at risk for developing psychiatric disorders at higher rates than the general population. This is due to interweaving influences based on a person's biology, psychology, and environment.

Slide 83

People with IDD frequently have a host of health related problems. As a group, persons with IDD have an increased prevalence of brain damage and seizure disorders.

At least 25% of all causes of IDD are known to be associated with biological abnormalities that affect the brain and often affect other body systems. Seizure disorders are increased proportionately as the level of IDD becomes more severe.

Some genetic syndromes associated with IDD are related to increased risk for certain psychiatric disorders (e.g., mood and anxiety disorders in persons with autism and Down syndrome). Some genetic syndromes as well as some psychiatric disorders can have a genetic predisposition (family history).

As a group, there is a greater prevalence of physical illnesses such as sensory deficits or disorders such as Autism, congenital heart disease, and gastrointestinal disorders. Additionally, they are at risk for medical and psychiatric misdiagnoses.

It is important to identify an individual's biological vulnerabilities as this offers opportunities to design and implement appropriate interventions.

Slide 84

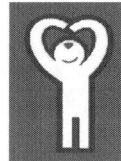

Vulnerability Factors

Vulnerability factors for psychiatric disorders:

Psychological

- Rejection/deprivation/abuse
- Life events/separations/losses
- Poor problem-solving/coping strategies
- Social/emotional/sexual vulnerabilities
- Poor self-acceptance/low self-esteem
- Devaluation/disempowerment

A person with IDD is often excluded from normative activities experienced by the general population (e.g., sport activities, parties). He/she may have to endure stigmatizing perceptions and negative social reactions and comments made by others.

Over-dependence, lack of confidence, poor self identity, or low self-esteem are characteristic in this population.

People with IDD have prolonged exposure to negative social conditions such as :

Labeling – People with IDD are vulnerable to experiencing psychologically devastating labels such as "retard" which create a perception of inferiority, difference, and exclusion.
Rejection and social disruption – People with IDD are often socially rejected or neglected by their peers, and feelings of loneliness are common.
Segregation – This can have severe psychological negative impacts. Segregation occurs across the lifespan from school through adulthood.
Restricted Opportunities –The majority of people with IDD will not have the usual opportunities for a rewarding life. For example, the vast majority will not have romantic relationships, will not marry, and will not experience parenthood.
Victimization – People with IDD are at risk for physical, sexual, and emotional abuse

Slide 85

Vulnerability Factors

Vulnerability factors for psychiatric disorders:

Social

- Negative attitudes/expectations
- **Stigmatization/prejudice/social exclusion**
- Poor supports/relationships/networks
- **Inappropriate environments/services**
- Financial/legal disadvantages

People with IDD are often socially isolated or do not have social networks that are common in the general population. Their social networks are usually made up of family members and caregivers ("artificial friendships").

These individuals are less likely to have natural developing friendships and thus identify staff as friends. This can be problematic because a staff member who has become a "significant other" may leave and the individual may feel repeatedly rejected and/or experience a significant loss.

Due to lack of experience in social situations people with IDD are vulnerable to being taken advantage of sexually, financially, and in many other ways. This is partly because the person is taught to comply and can be easily intimidated and/or coerced. Additionally, in many cases they would appreciate the attention, even when it's inappropriate.

The person with IDD who has a poor self image or low self-esteem may have a life that, by comparison to others, may feel unhappy, unsuccessful, and defeated.

Slide 86

Vulnerability Factors

Vulnerability factors for psychiatric disorders:

Family

- Diagnostic/bereavement issues
- **Life-cycle transitions/crises**
- Stress/adaptation to disability
- **Limited social/community networks**
- Difficulties "letting go"

The reaction of families to having an individual with a disability can be a risk factor, combined with other variables, in the development of psychiatric disorders. When parents give birth to a child who has a disability, they generally go through a bereavement process.

Individuals with IDD and their families go through a series of life transitions, and each one of these transitional stages can lead to a crisis situation. Some of these life transitions are :

-- identification of giving birth to a person with IDD
-    - beginning school
-    - being surpassed by younger siblings
-    - transitioning out of school
-    - being in the adult world
-- onset of psychiatric disorder
-- death of parents

Parents sometimes have difficulty in "letting go" and can tend to over-protect.

MODULE I

Slide 87

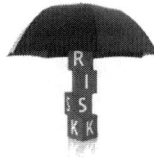

References: Module I

Accardo, P. & Capute, A. (1998). Mental retardations. *Mental Retardation and Developmental Disability Reviews, 4*, 2-5.

American Psychiatric Association. (2013). *Diagnostic and statistical manual of mental disorders* (5th ed.). Washington, DC: Author.

Ashley, S, & Clarren, S.K. (1999). *Diagnostic guide for FAS and related conditions: The 4-digit diagnostic code* (2nd ed.). Seattle, WA: University of Washington Press.

Carter, W. and Wehby, J. (2003). Job performance of transition-age youth with emotional and behavioral disorders. *Exceptional Children, 69*, 449-465.

Corbett, J.A.(1979). Psychiatric morbidity and mental retardation. In F.E. James, & R.P. Smith (Eds.), *Psychiatric illness and mental handicap* (pp. 11-23). London: Gaskill Press.

DiCicco-Bloom, E., Lord, C., Zwaigenbaum, L., Courchesne, E., Dager, S.R.,… Young, L.J.. (2006). The developmental neurobiology of autism. *The Journal of Neuroscience, 26*(26), 6897-6906.

Dykens, E. M., Hodapp, R. M. & Finucane, B. M. (2000). *Genetics and mental retardation syndromes: A new look at behavior and interventions.* Baltimore: Brookes.

Einfeld, S. L., & Aman, M. G. (1995). Issues in the taxonomy of psychopathology in children and adolescents with mental retardation. *Journal of Autism and Developmental Disorders, 25*, 143-167.

Einfeld, S.L., & Tonge, B.J. (1996). Population prevalence of psychopathology in children and adolescents with intellectual disability: II. Epidemiological findings. *Journal of Intellectual Disability Research,40*, 99-109.

Einfeld, S. & Emerson, E. (2009). *Intellectual disability. Rutter's child and adolescent psychiatry* (5th ed.). Oxford, U.K.: Blackwell Publishing.

Engel, G.L. (1980). The clinical application of the biopsychosocial model. *American Journal of Psychiatry, 137*, 535–544.

Finegan, J. (1998). Study of behavioral phenotypes: Goals and methodological concerns. *American Journal of Medical Genetics (Neuropsychiatric Genetics), 81*, 148-155.

Fletcher, R., Loschen, E., Stavrakaki, C., & First, M. (Eds.). (2007). *Diagnostic manual – Intellectual disability (DM-ID): A clinical guide for diagnosis of mental disorders in persons with intellectual disability.* Kingston, NY: NADD Press.

Flint, J., & Yule, W. (1994). Behavioural phenotypes. In Rutter, M.R., Taylor, E., and Hersov, L. (Ed.), *Child and adolescent psychiatry* (pp. 666-687). Oxford: Blackwell Scientific.

Goldberg, D. (2001). Vulnerability factors for common mental illnesses. *British Journal of Psychiatry, 178*(40), 69-71.

Government of Canada (2015). Statistics Canada. Retrieved on February 2015 from http://www.statcan.gc.ca/tables-tableaux/sum-som/l01/cst01/demo02a-eng.html .

Hagberg, B. & Witt-Engerstrom, I. (1986). Rett syndrome: A suggested staging system for describing impairment profile with increasing age towards adolescence. *American Journal of Medical Genetics, 24* (1), 4759.

Harrison, P.L., & Oakland, T. (2000). *Adaptive behavior assessment system*. San Antonio, TX: The Psychological Corporation.

Hartley, S.L. & McLean, W.E. (2009). Depression in adults with mild intellectual disability: the role of stress, attributions, and coping. *American Journal of Intellectual and Developmental Disabilities,* (114(3), 147-160.

Heiman, T., & Margalit, M. (1998). Loneliness, depression and social skills among students with mild mental retardation in special education and in mainstreamed classes. *Journal of Special Education, 32 (3),* 154 - 163.

Hobden, K.L., & LeRoy, B.W. (2009). Assessing mental health concerns in individuals with intellectual disabilities. *NADD Bulletin, 11* (3), 45-48.

Kent, L., Evans, J, Paul, M, & Sharp, M. (1999). Comorbidity of autistic spectrum disorders in children with Down syndrome. *Developmental Medicine & Child Neurology, 41*(3), 153-158.

McEvoy, R., Rogers, S., and Pennington, B. (2006) Executive function and social communication deficits in young autistic children. *Journal of Child Psychology and Psychiatry,* 34(4), 563-578.

Menolascino, F. J. (1977). *Challenges in mental retardation: Progressive ideology and services.* New York: Behavioral Publications.

National Core Indicators Adult Consumer Survey 2012-13 Final Report. (2014). National Association of State Directors of Developmental Disabilities Services and the Human Services Research Institute. Retrieved from www.nationalcoreindicators.org.

National Down Syndrome Society (2012). *Down Syndrome Facts.* Retrieved September, 2013 from http://www.ndss.org/Down-Syndrome/Down-Syndrome-Facts/

Consumer Outcomes Final Report 2010-2011 NCI Adult Consumer Survey Data, August 2012. Alexandria, VA: National Core Indicators.

O'Brien, G. & Yule, W. (1995). Why behavioural phenotypes? In G. O'Brien & W. Yule (Eds.), *Behavioural Phenotypes* (pp. 1-23). London: Mac Keith Press.

Royal College of Psychiatrists. (2001). *DC–LD: Diagnostic criteria for psychiatric disorders for use with adults with learning disabilities/mental retardation.* London: Gaskell Royal College of Psychiatrists.

Schalock, R.L., Borthwick-Duffy, S.A., Bradley, V.J., Buntix, W.H.E., Coulter, D.L., Craig, E.M.,…Yeager, M.H.(2010). *Intellectual disability: Definition, classification, and systems of support.* Washington, D.C.: American Association on Intellectual and Developmental Disabilities.

Simonoff, E., Bolton, P. & Rutter, M. (1998). Genetic perspectives on mental retardation. In J. A. Burack, R. M. Hodapp, & E. Zigler (Eds.), *Handbook of mental retardation and development* (pp. 41-79). Cambridge: Cambridge University Press.

Sparrow, S.S., Cicchetti, D.V., & Balla, D.A. (2005). Vineland Adaptive Behavior Scales, Second Edition (Vineland™-II). London, U.K.: AGS Publishing/Pearson Assessments.

Streissguth, A., Barr, H., Kogan, J., & Bookstein, F. *(1996). Understanding the occurrence of secondary disabilities in clients with Fetal Alcohol Syndrome (FAS) and Fetal Alcohol Effects (FAE).* Seattle, WA: University of Washington.

Streissguth, A., Bookstein, F.L., Barr, H.M., Sampson, P., O'Malley, K., Kogan Young, J. (2004). Risk factors for adverse life outcomes in fetal alcohol syndrome and fetal alcohol effects. *Developmental and Behavioral Pediatrics,* 25 (4), 228-238

Streissguth, A. & Kanter, J. (1997).*The challenge of fetal alcohol syndrome: Overcoming secondary disabilities.* Seattle, WA: University of Washington Press.

United States Census Bureau (2010). United States Census 2010. Retrieved March, 2014, from http://www.census.gov/2010census/#panel-4

Zigler, E. & Bennett-Gates, D. (1999). *Personality development in individuals with mental retardation.* Cambridge: Cambridge University Press.

MODULE I

M
O
D
U
L
E

I

Building on the Basics: Understanding Assessment Practices in Dual Diagnosis

Slide 1

Module II

Building on the Basics:
Understanding Assessment
Practices in Dual Diagnosis

Slide 2

CONCEPTUAL MODELS
RELATED TO BEHAVIORAL
PROBLEMS :

AN INTEGRATED ASSESSMENT
APPROACH

In assessing an individual who has IDD, it is important to identify the reasons why the individual is exhibiting behavioral problems. The question is often raised as to whether the maladaptive behavior is related to the person having an intellectual disability or related to the person having a mental illness. This is a false dichotomy as it is usually not just one causal relationship. Also, there may be other co-morbidities that contribute to the behavioral problem.

All potential problem areas and causes of the problem must be addressed by conducting an integrated assessment procedure.

Slide 3

> **This module includes content related to Conceptual Models Related to Behavior Problems: Integrative Approach, Functional Assessment of Behavior, and Assessment and Diagnostic Practices.**

Slide 4

Learning Objectives

- Articulate the elements of behavioral, medical, communication, and physical model of problem behavior
- List possible functions of challenging behavior
- Describe what is meant by ABCs of behavior
- Understand the considerations of and steps for a functional assessment
- Describe the best practice in assessment and diagnosis
- List the components and importance of the Integrative Model
- Describe the diagnostic principles for completing a psychiatric diagnosis in a person with IDD
- Describe why medical causes of problem behavior are often under-diagnosed
- Summarize the importance of obtaining past and present medical history as it relates to problem behavior
- Describe three medical conditions that can present as psychiatric issues/behavioral problems
- Articulate the importance of medical assessments in the assessment process
- Provide three examples of medical conditions that contribute to maladaptive behavior.

Slide 5

An On-going Case Study

Cal is a Caucasian man in his late 20s (date of birth April 26, 1992) with diagnoses of moderate intellectual disability and Autism Spectrum Disorder. He has a history of seizures, but is not currently treated for his seizure disorder, and there are no seizures observed at the current time. Cal is a fun person; he is very physical and has a silly sense of humor. He has some spoken language, and also communicates through action. He likes staying active, and while he lives in a group home setting, he also has a very involved family. He attends a day program.

MODULE II

Slide 6

Conceptual Models Related to Behavioral
Problems

Five Conceptual Models:

1. Medical Model

2. Communication Model

3. Behavioral Model

4. Psychiatric Model

5. Integrative Model (1-4)

When we think of problem behaviors in people with IDD, we often look for the etiology or reason why an individual's behavior is maladaptive. There are generally four schools of thought that are associated with maladaptive behaviors. These are medical models, communication models, behavioral models, and psychiatric models.

NADD has generally encouraged use of a fifth model, that being the integrative model. The integrative model assesses the dynamic influence of the previously mentioned four models to arrive at a multi-modal or integrative model. Often, there are multiple determinants that influence the expression of maladaptive behaviors. The integrative model assesses these various "pieces" and puts the clinical puzzle together as a whole.

A bio-psycho-social framework considers the multiple determinants and how each may contribute to the function of behavior. An integrative model provides a person-centered method of assessment.

Slide 7

Conceptual Models Related to
Behavioral Problems

1. Medical Model

- **Problem behaviors are exhibited because of co-existing medical problems**

- Assessment of potential medical problems involves conducting a full medical work-up

- **Treatment focuses on addressing the underlying medical problem**

Health disorders in people with IDD frequently differ from those encountered in the general population in terms of prevalence, age of onset, rate of progression, degree of severity, and presenting manifestations. These disorders are also more likely to be multiple and complex in those with IDD. (Haveman et al., 2009)

Medical conditions can mask as behavioral problems or psychiatric conditions. A person may "act out" as a way to express discomfort from a medical condition.

A full medical work up should be part of a mental health assessment process. Medical conditions should be assessed before looking at other causes of problem behaviors.

MODULE II

Slide 8

Conceptual Models Related to
Behavioral Problems

2. Communication Model

- Views behavioral problems as reflecting "challenging behaviors" in persons who have deficits in language skills

- Treatment – teach communication skills

- Assessment focuses on evaluation of skills, deficits and communicative intent.

Individuals with IDD often come from backgrounds that are impoverished of life-enriching experiences, especially in the area of communication.

Maladaptive behavior can be an attempt to communicate. Limited verbal repertoires reduce a person's ability to express feelings and communicate what he or she wants verbally, leading to behavioral attempts to communicate. For example, a person who has an IDD may experience the stress of an office visit. Without the verbal repertoire to express his or her discomfort verbally and indicate he or she wishes to leave, the person must rely on attempts to communicate physically through what could be perceived as aggressive behavior.

Slide 9

> ### Conceptual Models Related to Behavioral Problems
>
> ### 3. Behavioral Model
>
> - Problem behaviors are viewed according to learning principles
>
> - Assessment identifies the antecedent and consequences of the problematic behavior
>
> - Treatment focuses on changing or eliminating behavior though behavioral approaches
>
> - Does not usually identify people's needs/emotions.
>
> ster, Woll & Kuser, 1988

In the traditional behavioral model, the problem behavior is studied and then the environment is manipulated in such a way as to increase, decrease, or maintain the behavior. The problem or, as it is otherwise called, the target behavior is described, and then the antecedents and/or the consequences of the behavior are examined. This is known as the ABC approach.

The behavioral model is used extensively in the developmental disability field. Traditionally, the focus is on changing an unwanted behavior to a behavior that is more appropriate. The behavioral approach does not usually address people's feelings or emotions that are associated with the behavior. Rather, the focus of treatment is simply to change the behavior.

MODULE

II

Slide 10

4. Psychiatric Model

- Views problem behavior as a possible manifestation of a mental disorder

- Presentation of problem behaviors may be associated with a psychiatric disorder

- Assessment based on a bio-psycho-social model

- Treatment focuses on underlying psychiatric disorders

The psychiatric model essentially mirrors the medical model. The clinician identifies psychopathology in the individual, i.e., identification of a specific psychiatric disorder. The manifestation of the psychiatric disorder, for example sleep disturbance or loss of interest in preferred activities, is viewed as a manifestation of the identified psychiatric disorder. The treatment focuses on the underlying psychiatric disorder.

In the psychiatric model the first line of treatment typically would include a specific medication treatment or psychiatric intervention associated with a particular psychiatric diagnosis.

Slide 11

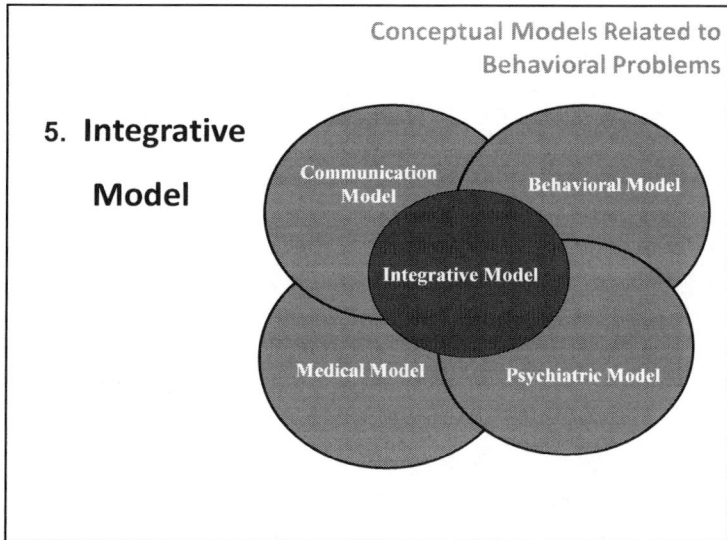

Conceptual Models Related to Behavioral Problems

5. **Integrative Model**

Communication Model

Behavioral Model

Integrative Model

Medical Model

Psychiatric Model

The integrative model assesses the individual's communication skills, assesses whether the individual is displaying maladaptive behaviors associated with learned behaviors, assesses the individual's medical conditions, and assesses whether the individual has a psychiatric disorder.

The integrative model assesses the dynamic overlapping influences and, after a comprehensive bio-psychosocial assessment, arrives at an integrative approach with regard to assessment and diagnosis.

Multiple determinants of problem behaviors are common in persons with IDD. Therefore, a multi-dimensional approach is critically important in conducting a comprehensive assessment in persons with IDD.

Positive Behavior Supports is one model that integrates the four aspects proposed in the integrated model: medical/biological considerations, psychiatric considerations, communication considerations, and behavior considerations. A PBS approach includes:

Functional Assessment
Comprehensive Intervention
Focus on quality of life and wellness   (Carr & Sidener, 2002)

PBS is discussed in detail in Module VII

MODULE II

Slide 12

Type of Model	Medical	Communication	Behavioral	Psychiatric
		The Relationship of Challenging Behavior and IDD		
Assessment	Medical Evaluation by primary care physician	Standardized administered measure of expressive language	Functional Analysis	DM-ID
Problem Identification	Constipation	Speech and language impairment	Function/ Need being met through behavior	Affective disorder, mania
Treatment	Medication for Bowel Movement (Laxative)	Functional communication skill training	Addressing unmet need, supporting appropriate behavior	Medication treatment, psychotherapy

In Cal's case, we conducted a bio-psychosocial assessment employing the integrative model. Therefore, we assessed the medical, communication, behavioral, and psychiatric domains. Each domain involved an assessment of the problem followed by a treatment protocol that corresponded to the medical, behavioral, communication, and psychiatric aspects of the problem.

It is very important to conduct this assessment within an interdisciplinary framework. As such, a holistic perspective is maintained throughout the assessment and treatment process.

Outcome: Cal has made significant improvement. His sleep and appetite are at normal levels. There has been a significant decrease in intensity and frequency of challenging behaviors.

Slide 13

Cal R.

Cal does engage in some problem behaviors that can be severe at times, and has caused injury to staff persons. His team recommended that a Functional Assessment be completed to gain a better understanding of his support needs, as there is a clear need to change his behavior as it interferes with community access and is a risk to the health of others.

In this case illustration, Cal is exhibiting a host of problems. One cannot determine from the information provided if Cal's problems are derived from a medical condition, communication impairment, learned behavior, or a psychiatric disorder.

The clinician needs to assess all the domains that may be influencing the problem behaviors. What could be contributing to, instigating, or triggering the maladaptive behaviors of SIB (Self-Injurious Behavior) and property destruction?

M
O
D
U
L
E

I
I

Slide 14

```
Functional Assessment of Problem Behavior

         The Function of Behavior
Behaviors may persist because the
    individual...
 • Enjoys the sensory experience – it feels better,
   satisfies a need or impulse (internal triggers,
   internal rewards)
 • Escapes or avoids demands or things he or she
   doesn't like to do
 • Gains attention from others
 • Obtains tangible items or opportunities – access
   to something he or she prefers
```

Professionals describe the possible functions in different ways and this outline avoids using a single word, but does organize around the four major categories highlighted in much of the literature:

• Tangibles
• Attention
• Escape
• Sensory – or as many refer to it – automatic reinforcement. In describing this category we try to emphasize that the behavior is generally triggered by internal stimuli and the reinforcing consequences also tend to be internal.

Slide 15

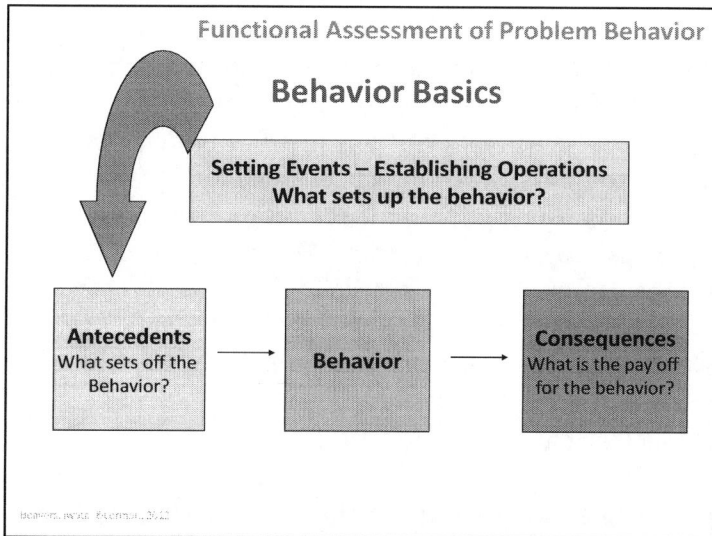

This is a visual representation of the A-B-C of behavior and categories we described above.

Slide 16

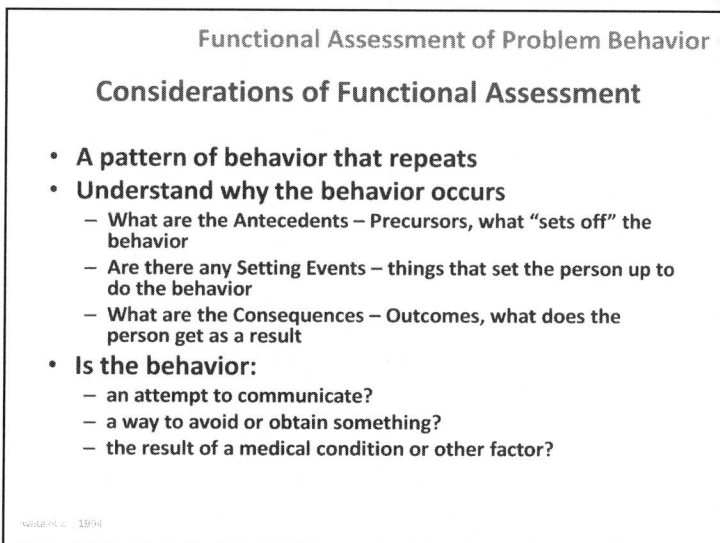

The slide introduces FBA, which is a way to understand the function of the behavior. The goal is to figure out what purpose a behavior serves for the individual; in other words, what makes it rewarding for them.

The big difference between understanding function of a behavior and traditional interpretations of behavior is from what perspective the behavior is viewed. Direct support professionals and clinicians need to understand the behavior through the eyes of the person who engages in it, rather than talking about the problems it causes for other people. Most of the time people talk about the behavior as inappropriate or inconvenient. For the person, it meets a need that he or she does not get in other ways.

This perspective is helpful through the remainder of the section.

The main points to learn are:

- Direct support professionals and clinicians need to focus on an observable behavior; something that they can see the person doing.
- There are basic elements that need to be understood and investigated in order to understand behavior. These include Antecedents and Consequences, which are discussed further in this section.
- Behavior can meet the needs of a person and can make sense from the person's perspective. Direct support professionals and clinicians need to be able to identify what need the person is attempting to meet and if the behavior is the most appropriate, effective way the person can meet the need.

Slide 17

> # Cal R.
>
> One of the main concerns is that when he is in parking lots, he must search through the parking lot and find out if there are any convertibles. If he is blocked from completing the search, he will become very aggressive and essentially do whatever it takes to do a thorough search, even if it is a huge lot. His family reports that they simply avoided any large parking lot of any type while he lived at home. He does love convertibles, and has a collection of small convertible cars, and loves seeing them on tv. Numerous persons have referred to this as OCD, though he does not have a formal diagnosis of OCD. There is an ongoing debate, at time acrimonious, between care providers & family who consider this OCD and care providers & family who consider this a symptom of ASD.

From Slide 14 – using the four possible reasons listed about why a behavior might persist, can you develop a hypothesis about Cal's behavior. Is it one of the examples listed below, or could it be something else?

Is it an attempt to communicate?
Is it a way to avoid or obtain something?
Is it the result of a medical condition or other factor?

M
O
D
U
L
E

I
I

Slide 18

> ### Functional Assessment of Problem Behavior
>
> #### The Steps to a Functional Assessment
>
> - Describe what the target behavior is; the operational definition
> - Interview the person or care providers
> - Observe the person to see what else might be happening
> - Use the interview and observation to make some guesses about the antecedents and consequences
> - Identify antecedents, setting events, and consequences (outcomes)
> - Look for patterns to identify function

Now we make the transition. Before we start using antecedent-based interventions, it is important to know what the function is and which antecedents to address.

Slide 19

> ### Functional Assessment of Problem Behavior
>
> #### Look for Patterns
>
> - The same type of triggers tend to set the behavior off
> - People respond in similar ways to maintain the behavior, the person gets the same kind of outcome
> - Setting events (establishing operations) make behavior more likely to occur when trigger is present.
> - The behavior doesn't have to happen every time the trigger is present but work enough to make the behavior "worth it" for the individual.

Setting events and triggers can act as cues for the person to engage in a specific behavior.

The identification of patterns of triggers and responses assists in the functional assessment of behavior by helping to identify the conditions under which a specific behavior is likely to occur. If similar conditions lead to similar responses with high frequency, the conditions to analyze the function are present.

Slide 20

Functional Assessment of Problem Behavior

Go to the Experts
Involving direct caregivers in plan development
- **Staff often work closest to and spend most time with people**
- **Encourage contributions, observations, hypotheses, ideas, intervention strategies**
- **Staff can identify trends and missing puzzle pieces that managers and behaviorists often cannot**
- **Foster control and confidence**
- **Promote participation and involvement in planning**
- **Consider opinions and answer questions**
- **Provide ongoing support and guidance**

MODULE II

Direct support professionals and caregivers are the people who generally spend the most time with the person. They can have valuable and insightful contributions to make about observations of the person, ideas around why the behavior occurs and possible intervention strategies based on their knowledge and experience with the person.

The benefits of including direct support professionals and caregivers:
- Opportunity for staff to take ownership in planning for the individuals they support
- More likely to follow plans and strategies if involved in development
- Increases staff self-efficacy in following plans, or implementing strategies
- Greater consistency
- Staff learn to be more observant & more comfortable contributing information
- More accurate and useful information will emerge
- Individuals will associate staff with progress and challenging behavior will decrease

Slide 21

> # Cal R.
>
> A Functional Assessment of Behavior was completed by a consultant that closely focused on the issues around parking lots and convertibles. It was determined that once Cal finds a convertible, he will continue on with the prior activities (i.e., he does not need to find a second convertible, though if it is a small parking lot he may briefly look for a second one). Additionally, if no convertible is found in the entire lot, he will continue with prior activities. This information was shared with his primary care physician at an appointment, which was also attended by team members and the consultant who completed the FA.

Slide 22

> # Cal R. - The outcome
>
> The DM-ID (based on the DSM-IV-TR) was reviewed. At that point, the determination was made that there was no evidence of OCD, and that this pattern of behavior was a symptom of the ASD, and treatment was developed from a perspective informed by ASD, including the use of Social Stories and Structured Teaching.

Slide 23

> ### Exercise
>
> **Review the case information on Slides 17 and 21 for Cal. List 2 ways staff involvement was instrumental in the process.**

If necessary, provide an example such as "Staff should participate."

Slide 24

> BEST PRACTICES
>
> IN
>
> ASSESSMENT AND DIAGNOSTIC
>
> PROCEDURES

Slide 25

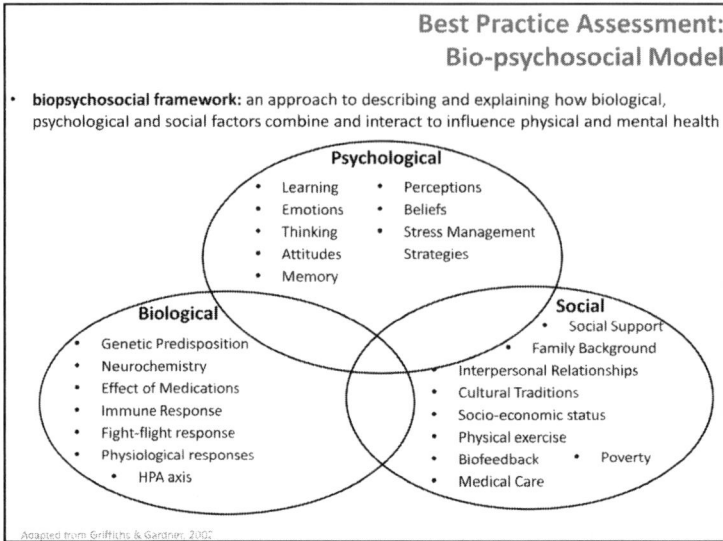

Best Practice Assessment: Bio-psychosocial Model

- **biopsychosocial framework:** an approach to describing and explaining how biological, psychological and social factors combine and interact to influence physical and mental health

Psychological
- Learning   • Perceptions
- Emotions   • Beliefs
- Thinking   • Stress Management
- Attitudes   Strategies
- Memory

Biological
- Genetic Predisposition
- Neurochemistry
- Effect of Medications
- Immune Response
- Fight-flight response
- Physiological responses
    • HPA axis

Social
    • Social Support
    • Family Background
- Interpersonal Relationships
- Cultural Traditions
- Socio-economic status
- Physical exercise
- Biofeedback   • Poverty
- Medical Care

Adapted from Griffiths & Gardner, 2002

The biopsychosocial framework provides an integrated model of assessment. If we limit ourselves to a single way to try and understand the challenges posed in supporting a person with IDD/MI, we will miss the mark in most cases and fail to understand the true complex nature of needs. One of the philosophical difficulties we encounter in supporting this population is that many professionals only consider their specific discipline and professional training, and as such don't consider other ways to view the challenges of the person.

Exacerbating this is the fact that many assessment tools are based on the practices of a specific discipline. For example, a behavior analytic assessment tool may primarily ask questions leading to a functional assessment of behavior, considering setting events, discriminative stimuli, and maintaining consequences, but not delving into physiological events or asking why certain events have such a degree of salience. Similarly, a mental health assessment may fail to take into account the explanatory power of a person's culture. The bio-psychosocial assessment is an effort to address these types of problems by creating an assessment model that includes and embraces multiple disciplinary perspectives.

Slide 26

Best Practice of Biopsychosocial Model

1. Incorporates the effects of biomedical and psychological factors and how these influences interrelate.

2. Uses assessment information to guide selection of diagnostically based interventions.

Griffiths & Gardner 20..

Bio-psychosocial assessment specifically considers the factors listed on the prior slide. In a complex situations in supporting a person with IDD/MI, all of these factors overlap and inter-relate. For example, if a person takes a decongestant that cause insomnia (bio), gets very frustrated by being awake at night and copes by watching horror movies at high volume (psycho), and awakens family members leading to family stress (social), all three factors need to be considered in taking a comprehensive look at understanding these difficulties. The bio-psychosocial assessment model will guide subsequent design of intervention. In the example, all three areas would need to be considered, with both short- and long-term goals being of clinical necessity.

MODULE II

Slide 27

> Best Practice of Bio-psycho-social Model
>
> 3. **Identifies skills and related supports required by the individual to cope effectively with multiple biopsychosocial influences.**
>
> 4. **Proactive in focus.**
>
> 5. **Provides for translation of multiple modalities of influence in a common model.**
>
> Griffiths, Gardner 2002

The bio-psycho-social model identifies skill deficits as possible causes of behavior, anticipates needs, and makes accommodations for biomedical and psychological factors identified in assessment.

The bio-psycho-social model also considers the supports in place and the supports needed. Skills deficits, such as communication and stress management, are significant contributors to mental health challenges and related problems. Related supports are equally relevant.

A person's environment generally determines how severe a problem is perceived or becomes. Supports can buffer against a problem behavior or can assure an effective, rapid response to a mental health problem. Consider the example from the prior slide. Skills for self-management during nocturnal wakefulness are needed, as well as a quick end to the decongestant use. The bio-psycho-social model seeks to promote a proactive mode of addressing challenges by heading them off rather than reacting to a problem after it occurs. For mental health, the focus is always on increasing mental wellness, NADD's stated mission. The consideration is facilitated by considering biological, psychological, and social modalities of understanding within a single model.

Slide 28

Best Practice of Bio-psycho-social Model

6. **Provides an integrated multimodal treatment plan.**

7. **Recognizes that mental health consists of both the presence of personal contentment, and the relative absence of psychological distress.**

William K. Gardner 2003

The inclusion of different perspectives into a single model directly leads to an integrated multimodal treatment plan. Having a unified understanding of a person's support needs in a single assessment increases the likelihood of having a single plan of intervention and treatment, which will promote coordination of intervention and simplicity of support provision.

Finally, the bio-psycho-social model recognizes that mental health isn't just the absence of a disorder. It include the presence of positive emotion. In this framework, personal contentment is a valid consideration, as are other forms of mental wellness and positive experiences and character traits.

MODULE II

Slide 29

Best Practice Assessment:
Bio-psycho-social Model

1. Review Reports

2. Interview Family

3. Interview Care Provider

4. Direct Observation

5. Clinical Interview

A comprehensive assessment process involves gathering existing data and background information. Additionally, interviewing the individual as well as relevant others are also essential components of the assessment process. Making observations in the natural environments is also important.

Conducting a comprehensive assessment takes much more time than an assessment of a person from the general population. The interview with the client is important, but insufficient in conducting a comprehensive assessment.

The clinician first needs to get releases to obtain information from a variety of sources such as :
- School
- Foster Home / Group Home
- Residential Institutions
- Outpatient Mental Health Services
- Primary Care Physician
- Other

Slide 30

> ### Mental Health Assessment & Managing the Interview
>
> - **Obtain records in advance**
>   - School, medical, development and family
> - **Become familiar with collateral informants who attend the interview**
>   - Parents, care provider, service coordinators
> - **Understand that the assessment interview can be stressful for all involved**
>   - Interviewer will need to be alert for increased distress on part of the client
>
> Morrison & Grau, 2014

When completing a mental health assessment, there are a number of tips the interviewer would find helpful in completing the assessment process.

By obtaining records in advance of the assessment, the interviewer is able to review information and history pertinent to the current situation. It may also provide a more thorough history than the person is able to relate him- or herself.

Good sources of information are staff, caregivers, family members, etc. They likely spend the most time with the person and have a helpful knowledge of their history and current condition.

MODULE II

Slide 31

> ### Mental Health Assessment & Managing the Interview
>
> - **Assessment interview will likely take more time than with a neurotypical person**
> - **Examiner needs to use language that correlates with the expressive and receptive language skills of the client**
>   - Simple language
>   - Reflection
>   - Stay away from abstract concepts and analogies

When completing the mental health assessment, the clinician will want to be sure to:

- Use simple language, avoid jargon and slang
- Use reflection to ensure the accurate message is conveyed
- Avoid abstract concepts and comparisons. Language should be concrete and direct.

Slide 32

> ### Mental Health Assessment & Managing the Interview
>
> - **Watch for signs the person is trying to respond to questions in a way that will please the interviewer.**
>
> - **Parroting and perseverating habits may interfere with the accuracy of the responses.**
>
> - **Multiple assessment interviews may be needed to obtain a full assessment.**
>
> Thomson & Gong, 2013

People with IDD often want to please the interviewer and will answer questions in ways that are perceived to please.

People with IDD may repeat words and language they have heard but don't fully understand in an attempt to mask their disability.

Attention to detail may be difficult for the person in a prolonged interview. The clinician may want to break the interview into shorter sessions that are more manageable for the client with IDD.

Slide 33

> Mental Health Assessment
>
> I. Source of Information and Reason for Referral
>
> II. History of Presenting Problem and Past Psychiatric History
>
> III. Family Health History
>
> IV. Social and Developmental History

The purpose of an assessment is to identify the developmental, biological, psychological, and environmental factors that might be associated with precipitating and/or maintaining the maladaptive behavior.

It is important to obtain information from multiple sources. These assessments frequently require a multidisciplinary approach as there may be multiple factors at play and no one approach can truly develop the necessary holistic level of understanding.

As the person with IDD may have limitations with regard to communication skills, it is therefore important to rely on reports from others. These reports should convey current as well as historical information. Arriving at an understanding of why a particular maladaptive behavior has developed, or establishing whether there has been an apparent change in mood, mental state, or general well being, may be a considerable challenge to the person(s) conducting the assessment.

Inadequate assessment may lead to ill-informed interventions. Many factors must be considered in the assessment process: traumatic experience, living arrangements, education/employment status, goals, person-centered plans, modes of communication, etc.

Slide 34

> ### Mental Health Assessment
>
> I. **Source of Information and Reason for Referral**
>
> - **Who made the referral?**
>
> - **What is different from baseline behavior?**
>
> - **Why make the referral now?**

It is important to know who made the referral and the reason for the referral for the assessment. Unlike with the neurotypical person, referrals for mental health assessments are generally not made by the client but by care providers involved in the individual's life.

There are occasions where it has been determined that the actual problem does not primarily involve the person being referred, but instead the person or environment who referred the client for a mental health assessment.

The following questions should be asked :
- Who made the referral (i.e., agency, parent)?
- Why is the referral being made now?
- What is the presenting problem?
- What are the expectations of the referring source?
- What is the person's perception of the problem?

Slide 35

Mental Health Assessment

II. History of Presenting Problem and Past Psychiatric History

- How long has the problem occurred?
    - History of mental health treatment
    - Trauma history

The assessment process needs to include obtaining information regarding the history of the presenting problem. It is, therefore, important to obtain background history such as :

- Chronological history of problem
- Significant symptomology
- Precipitating factors

If the person has had a past psychiatric history, the assessment should include the following:

- Outpatient mental health services including diagnosis, therapies, medications, and response to treatment
- Inpatient mental health services including diagnosis, therapies, medications, and response to treatment

Slide 36

> **Mental Health Assessment**
>
> III. **Personal and Family Health History**
> - **Medical, psychiatric, and substance abuse history**
>
> - **Psychotropic medications**
>
> - **Medical conditions**
>   - **Genetic disorders**
>   - **Hypo/hyper thyroid condition**
>   - **Constipation**
>   - **Epilepsy**
>   - **Diabetes**
>   - **Gastrointestinal problem**

The assessment process needs to obtain information regarding personal and family health history. Medical conditions as well as mental health disorders can have a genetic predisposition. For example, affective disorders tend to have a genetic predisposition and therefore can be passed from one generation to another.

Physical illnesses are important differential diagnoses for most psychiatric presentations in people with IDD. People with IDD have a higher prevalence of physical illness compared to other population groups.

Full blood count, measures of thyroid, kidney and liver function, and blood glucose are important routine blood tests and should be ascertained as part of a comprehensive mental health assessment.

In fact, a physical health assessment should be conducted first in order to determine whether a behavioral problem is caused by a physical health problem.

Slide 37

> Mental Health Assessment
>
> IV. Social/Developmental History
>
> - Developmental milestones
> - Relevant school history
> - Work/vocational history
> - Current work/vocational status
> - Legal issues
> - Relevant family dynamics
> - Drug/alcohol history
> - Abuse history
>   (emotional/physical/sexual)
> - Trauma history

An important part of the assessment process is gathering information regarding a social and developmental history. Some of this information such as developmental milestones can be obtained from parents. Other information, can be obtained from other resources. The clinician may have to obtain records from various sources such as school and residential and/or day programs.

Research has indicated that the majority of people with IDD have experience some type of abuse, including sexual abuse. Therefore, obtaining information about abuse history is very important. This can be a delicate matter if family members or other significant others are suspected of the abuse. Depending on the level of functioning of the individual, the use of anatomical dolls, pictures, and other non-verbal forms of communication can be useful.

Slide 38

> ### Mental Health Assessment
>
> **Behavioral Status Review Reports**
>
>   A. **Recent Changes**
>
>   B. **Problem Behavior**
>
>   C. **Quality of Life Issues**

Conducting a mental health assessment with a person who has IDD is a very complex task. There are ways to assist in attempting to identify behavioral problems as well as the source of the problem. As noted previously, factors to consider in this portion of an assessment include but are not limited to: traumatic experience, employment/education status, living arrangements, goals, person centered plans, etc.

It is also useful to list the assets/positive aspects that are meaningful to the individual. These positive attributes not only have meaning but can promote the quality of life for the individual.

Slide 39

Behavioral Status: Recent Changes: A

Name: _____   Today's Date: _____

Date of last appointment: _____ Person completing this form _____

A.   Primary reason(s) for this consultation: _____

B.   Life changes that have occurred within the last six (6) months

	Yes	No	Comments
1. Moves			
2. Deaths of significant others			
3. Staff or teacher changes			
4. New roommates/classmates			
5. Problems			
6. Loss of friend, pet, family member			
7. Loss of key staff/teacher			
8. Evidence of a delayed grief reaction			
9. Change in employment, program or leisure activities			

C. Acute medical problems or changes in past medical condition since last visit:

_____

In this chart the clinician or care provider can indicate life changes that have occurred over the last 6 months. Any one of these items (1-9) can contribute to or somehow be related to a behavioral problem. In this chart we are looking at changes in the environment that may affect behavior.

Additionally, any changes in medical conditions can be associated with behavioral problems as noted in "C" on the chart above.

Slide 40

	C	A	E	N/A	Comments
Behavioral Status: **Problem Behavior: B**					
1. **Is aggressive**					
2. **Is self injurious**					
3. **Appears anxious**					
4. **Socially isolates self**					
5. **Is overactive**					
6. **Is under-active**					

<u>C</u>hronic: Person displays behavior on a daily basis, but severity may wax and wane

<u>A</u>cute: Behavior represents a dramatic change

<u>E</u>pisodic: Periods of disturbance and periods of normal functioning

<u>N/A</u>: Non-Applicable

This is another chart that can assist in the assessment process. In this chart we are looking at eleven areas that may be indicative, but not necessarily proof of a mental health disorder.

The clinician or care provider checks off whether the particular behavior is chronic, acute, episodic, or non-applicable.

When questioning regarding self-injury, the clinician must receive a detailed, precise description of the problem behavior, e.g., SIB – punching self with closed fist – vs – slapping ones face. Behaviors can be considerably different but may be reported in the same context unless the clinician asks for specific details about the behavior. Clarity around exactly what the behavior looks like is vital for accurate assessment.

MODULE II

Slide 41

Behavioral Status:
Problem Behavior: B (continued)

	C	A	E	N/A	Comments
7. Engages in ritualistic behavior, compulsions					
8. Has self-stimulatory behavior					
9. Steals					
10. Has tantrums					
11. Is impulsive					
12. OTHER (explain):					

Chronic: Person displays behavior on a daily basis, but severity may wax and wane

Acute: Behavior represents a dramatic change

Episodic: Periods of disturbance and periods of normal functioning

N/A: Non-Applicable

Beasley, Kroll, & Sovner 1992

The behavioral items provide yet another clue to the complex task of a mental health assessment for persons with IDD.

Slide 42

Behavioral Status:
Quality of Life Issues: C

Please list and explain the areas that he/she enjoys that promotes quality of life.

Family: _____

Friends: _____

Living Situation: _____

Leisure Activities: _____

Staff Relations: _____

Hobbies: _____

Work: _____

Other: _____

Beasley, Kroll, & Sovner 1992

The assessment process should also include listing the positive attributes, desires, and pleasurable activities of the individual. This can include not only activities enjoyed by the client but also important relationships involved in the individual's life.

Slide 43

In assisting with the complex challenge of conducting an assessment, it is very useful to obtain certain types of data.

- Physical health – Health problems are often associated with behavioral problems
- Sleep data – Problems with sleep can be indicative of a mental health problem
- Medication changes – These can have an adverse effect on behavior
- Eating patterns – A change in appetite can be indicative of a mental health problem
- Environmental changes – These can cause stress and lead to behavioral problems
- Mood charting – A change in mood can be indicative of a mental health disorder

Slide 44

\

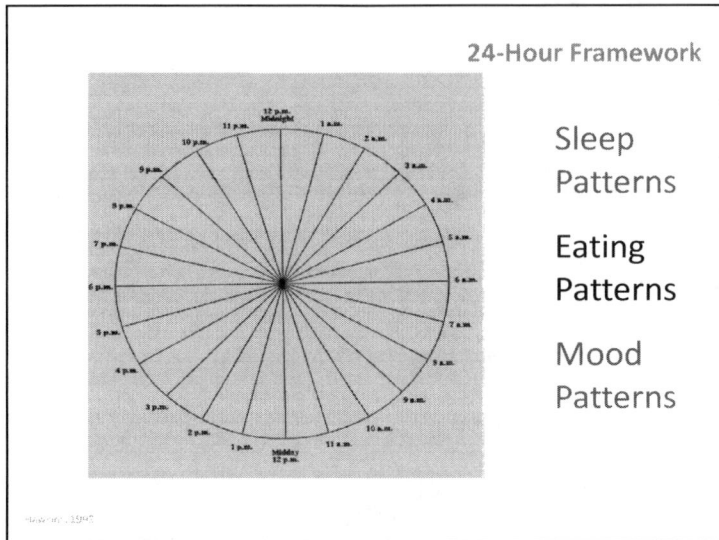

24-Hour Framework

Sleep
Patterns

Eating
Patterns

Mood
Patterns

There are an assortment of ways to collect data. The data collection process can change from agency to agency. Also, if the individual lives with his or her natural family, then a 24 hour pie chart as listed above may be a challenge.

The pie chart is based on a 24 hour period with charting for each hour. Another and perhaps easier method of charting sleep, eating, and mood patterns is to use a chart that indicates sleep, eating and mood on a daily basis rather than an hourly basis.

Slide 45

> ## Exercise
>
> Cal is a man with diagnoses of moderate intellectual disability and Autism Spectrum Disorder. He has a history of seizures, but is not currently treated for his seizure disorder and there are no seizures observed currently. A primary concern is that when he is in parking lots, he must search the entire lot to find any convertibles. If he is blocked from completing the search, he will become very aggressive and essentially do whatever it takes to do a thorough search regardless of the size of the lot. His family reports that they avoided any large parking lots while he lived at home. Numerous people have referred to this as OCD, though there is no formal diagnosis. There is an ongoing debate, at times bitter, between care providers, who consider this a symptom of ASD, and family who, consider this OCD.

ACTIVITY:

1) What data needs to be collected to assist with planning for appropriate supports?

2) What interventions can we put in place for Cal immediately while we gather more information?

MODULE II

Slide 46

> Myth: Individuals with IDD Cannot Have a
> Verifiable Mental Health Disorder
>
> **PREMISE:**
> **Maladaptive behaviors are a function of IDD**
>
> **REALITY:**
> The full range of psychiatric disorders can be
> represented in persons with IDD
>
> **DIAGNOSTIC IMPLICATIONS:**
> **Psychiatric diagnosis can be made using the**
> **DM-ID, DSM-5 records, service providers, family**
> **input, and client interview**

This myth is based on the historical notion that behavioral problems in people with IDD are directly associated with having the condition of IDD.

The reality is that the full range of psychiatric conditions that are expressed in the general population are also represented in persons with IDD. In fact, there is a higher prevalence rate of psychiatric disorders in persons with IDD as compared to the general population.

An appropriate diagnostic procedure is both complex and time consuming. It involves obtaining and gathering multiple sources of information. The use of either the DSM or DM-ID is needed.

Slide 47

Eight Diagnostic Principles For Recognizing
Psychiatric Disorders In
People with IDD

1. People with Intellectual/Developmental Disabilities suffer from the full range of psychiatric disorders.

2. Psychiatric disorders usually present as maladaptive behavior.

3. The origin of psychopathology has multiple etiologies.

Adapted from Sovner & Hurley, 1986

1. Psychiatric disorders in people with IDD are considered to be at a higher prevalence rate than in the general population. This includes disorders in children, adolescents, adults, as well as older adults.
2. Behavioral problems or maladaptive behaviors are often associated with the manifestation of a psychiatric disorder. This is different than what occurs in the general population, as people with IDD usually manifest a psychiatric disorder through observations of their behavior and these behavior are often maladaptive.
3. There can be internal as well as external contributing factors to the origin of a psychiatric disorder in a person with IDD. There are interwoven influences from a bio-psycho-social-family perspective.

Slide 48

> Eight Diagnostic Principles For Recognizing
> Psychiatric Disorders
> In People with IDD (continued)
>
> 4. **An acute psychiatric disorder may present as an exaggeration of longstanding maladaptive behavior**
>
> 5. **Maladaptive behavior rarely occurs alone**
>
> 6. **The severity of the problem is not diagnostically relevant**
>
> Adapted from Sovner 1987

4. Maladaptive behaviors that previously existed may increase in frequency and intensity during the onset of a mental illness. For example, an individual might have a low rate of mild Self-Injurious Behavior, but during the time of stress, the frequency and intensity of this behavior can escalate to a high level. This may be at a time when a psychiatric diagnosis is made.

5. Generally, the occurrence of repeated maladaptive behaviors in a person with IDD is a clear clue to the presence of a psychiatric disorder. People with IDD usually don't have serious and persistent maladaptive behaviors as part of the condition of having IDD. Rather these maladaptive behaviors are more likely to be a manifestation of a psychiatric disorder. Therefore, maladaptive behaviors rarely occur alone.

6. The severity of a maladaptive behavior, such as an act of aggression, does not lead to a mental health diagnosis. In fact, aggression is a non-specific behavior that may or may not be related to a diagnosis. (Sovner & Hurley, 1989)

Slide 49

> Eight Diagnostic Principles For Recognizing
> Psychiatric Disorders
> In People with IDD (continued)
>
> 7. The clinical interview alone is rarely diagnostic.
>
> 8. It is very difficult to diagnose psychotic disorders in people with very limited verbal skills.
>
> Adapted from Sovner & Hurley, 1983

7. Interviewing the client is a condition of, but insufficient for, a comprehensive diagnostic assessment. People with IDD tend to "acquiesce" as they want to please the interviewer. Also, people at the lower end of the intellectual range may not have the expressive and receptive language skills or may have limited vocabulary which complicates engagement in a meaningful interview. Multiple sources of data collection are therefore necessary to obtain relevant information that will assist in the assessment and diagnostic process since communication deficits can create barriers to assessment interviews.

8. Psychotic disorders such as schizophrenia usually require the client to provide a self report of signs and symptoms. For example, the person would express experiencing hallucinations and delusions. These are internal states that are difficult if not impossible to observe. Therefore, verbal skills are helpful, if not essential, for the diagnosis of psychotic disorders. Hence the diagnosis of psychotic disorders becomes increasingly difficult to make with increasing degrees of IDD.

Slide 50

Barriers to Diagnosis and Treatment

15 Complicating Diagnostic Factors

1) **Diagnostic Overshadowing**
2) Problems with Poly pharmacy
3) **Communication Deficits**
4) Atypical Presentation of Psychiatric Disorders
5) **Limited Life Experiences**
6) Medical Conditions
7) **Acquiescence**

8) Learned Behavior
9) **Aggression and SIB (self-injurious behavior)**
10) Sensory Impairment
11) **Behavioral Overshadowing**
12) Medication Masking
13) **Episodic Presentation**
14) Division of Services
15) **Lack of Expertise**

Diagnosis of mental illness in people with an IDD can be complicated by a number of factors as indicated above.

Slide 51

Barriers to Diagnosis and Treatment

Complicating Diagnostic Factors (1-3)

1) Diagnostic Overshadowing

2) Problems with Poly Pharmacy

3) Communication Deficits

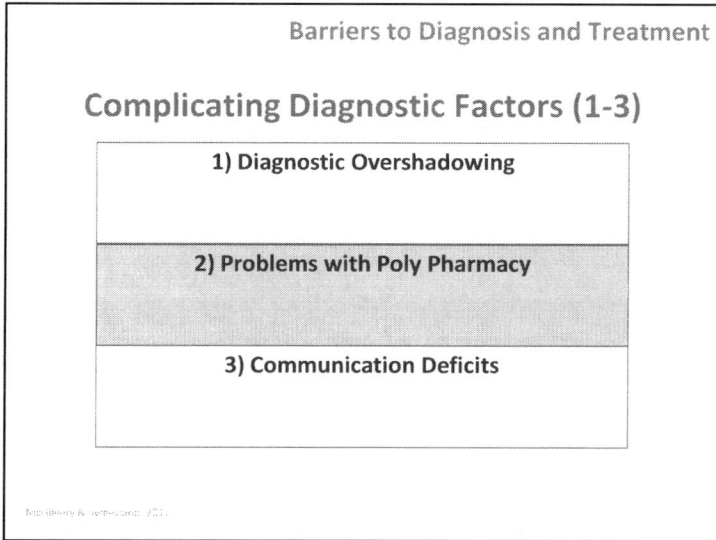

1) Diagnostic Overshadowing – Reiss, Leviton, and Szyszko (1982) developed the term diagnostic overshadowing to indicate the tendency to attribute many of the possible symptoms of a psychiatric disorder to the intellectual/developmental disability. For example, when a person with an IDD communicates being upset by "acting out," it can be defined as a behavioral challenge.

2) Problems with Poly Pharmacy – Individuals with IDD are sometimes on multiple medications and some are on multiple medications of the same class. That is to say they may be on multiple medications treating the same symptom. This can present medical, as well as behavioral problems. Some of the side effects of the medication can produce symptoms that are similar to a psychiatric disorder. For example, fatigue, confusion, agitation, lethargy, short attention span, or changes in sleep or appetite are common medication side effects. They are also symptoms of mental health disorders.

3) Communication Deficits – Individuals with IDD often have difficulty in expressive language skills. Additionally, they frequently come from backgrounds that are impoverished of life enriching experiences, especially in the area of communication. If the individual's verbal ability or insight is limited, that person is not likely to provide an accurate presentation of symptoms.

MODULE II

Slide 52

Barriers to Diagnosis and Treatment

Complicating Diagnostic Factors (4-6)

4) Atypical Presentation of Psychiatric Disorders

5) Limited Life Experiences

6) Medical Conditions

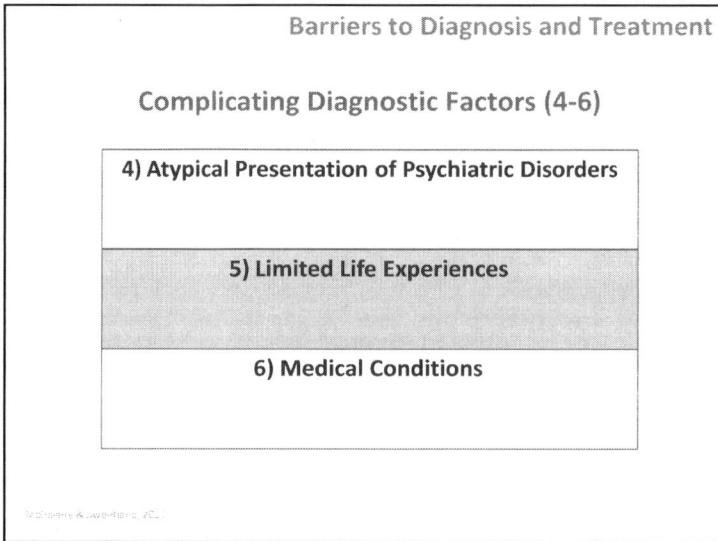

4) **Atypical Presentation of Psychiatric Disorders** – Persons with IDD may manifest a psychiatric symptom in a different way than a person from the general population. Often, the expression of a psychiatric disorder is through behavioral disturbances rather than through a self report of symptoms. It is not uncommon for a person with IDD to "act out" in a maladaptive manner, rather than give a self report of how he or she feels. Severe behavioral disturbances in the form of verbal or physical aggression is not uncommon and may be related to a psychiatric disorder. Therefore, observing behavior is very important rather than reliance on self report.

5) **Limited Life Experiences** - Due to a narrow range of life experiences, it may be difficult to detect some of the symptoms of a psychiatric disorder. For example, a typically developing individual with bipolar disorder who is in a manic phase may spend excessively and charge up credit cards or increase social activity, sometimes to an unsafe level. An individual with an intellectual disability may not have the financial resources for overspending, promiscuous relationships, travel, etc. Therefore, the diagnosis may be missed because the symptoms look different.

6) **Medical Conditions** – Medical conditions often co-occur with psychiatric disorders in persons with IDD. Medical conditions can mask psychiatric disorders; it is therefore very important to assess medical conditions as one of the first areas in conducting a mental health assessment. Limited communication skills make it difficult for the person to express pain and discomfort. Typical signs and symptoms of a mental health disorder can reflect signs and symptoms of a medical condition.

Slide 53

```
Barriers to Diagnosis and Treatment

Complicating Diagnostic Factors (7-9)

        7) Acquiescence

        8) Learned Behavior

    9) Aggression and SIB (self-Injurious Behavior)
```

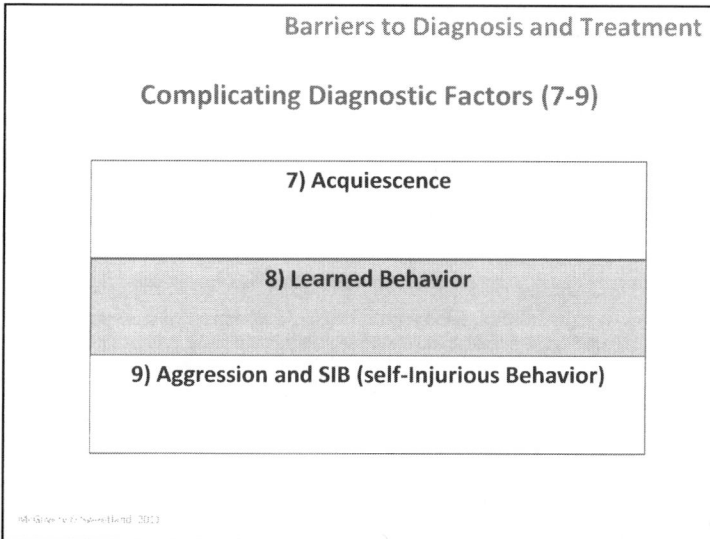

7) Acquiescence – Interviewing someone who has an intellectual disability and obtaining accurate information about the individual's symptoms can be confounded by an increased tendency for the person to agree quickly. The person may tell the clinician or care provider what he or she thinks the interviewer wants to hear or agree to things in order to avoid the risk of disapproval. The person may be more likely to report "yes" or "no" to all questions despite the true response.

8) Learned Behavior – An individual with IDD may exhibit behaviors that have been learned and modeled from others. For example, a person may begin a spitting behavior after observing and thus learning this behavior from another individual in the group home. A person may learn task avoidance behaviors from others in his or her environment. For example, at an adult group home for people with mild levels of IDD a person might refuse to do dishes when it's his or her turn; and this behavior may be modeled on others in the group home. This can be considered a secondary function of behavior.

9) Aggression and SIB – Self injurious behavior and aggression are often displayed by people with IDD. However, they are not diagnostically related to any one psychiatric diagnosis. SIB and aggressive behaviors can result from either internal or external triggers and setting events. For example, a person can display aggression or SIB associated with a specific psychiatric disorder such as mania or could display these behaviors associated with stress from the external environment.

Slide 54

> **Barriers to Diagnosis and Treatment**
>
> ### Complicating Diagnostic Factors (10-12)
>
> | 10) Sensory Impairment |
> |---|
> | 11) Behavioral Overshadowing |
> | 12) Medication Masking |
>
> McConkey & Sreenaras, 2013

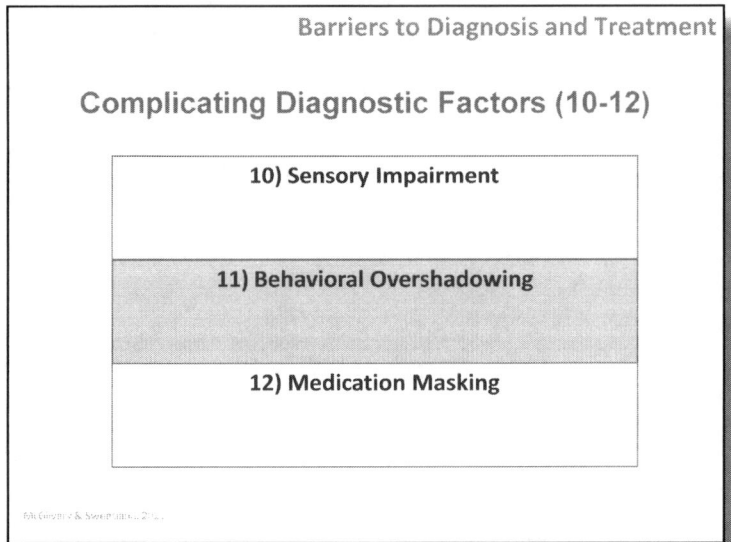

10) Sensory Impairment – It is important to consider whether the individual has any sensory impairments (sight, hearing, touch, etc.). For example, it is not usual for an individual who is totally blind to have disruptions in sleep. Therefore, diagnosing depression based on changes in sleep as one criterion, or diagnosing a sleep disorder in light of these disruptions, may be inaccurate. Similarly, it is not unusual for a person with a hearing impairment to become agitated with changes in a schedule because, not having heard the conversation about making new plans, the person finds the changes unexpected.

11) Behavioral Overshadowing – Behavioral Overshadowing refers to a tendency to identify psychopathology as learned behavior while failing to recognize it as an indicator of mental illness. For example, a person's behavioral challenges may be thought to be related to "task avoidance" rather than loss of motivation due to schizophrenia.

12) Medication Masking – The sedative effects of certain medications (e.g., typical antipsychotic medications) can suppress, or mask, the presence of significant mental health symptoms. For example, a person may be experiencing agitation related to depression but, due to limited communication skills, be unable to describe symptoms of their depression. If the person is prescribed a typical antipsychotic medication, the agitation may stop. However, the medication has not effectively treated the person's illness, and he or she may continue to suffer with symptoms of depression.

Slide 55

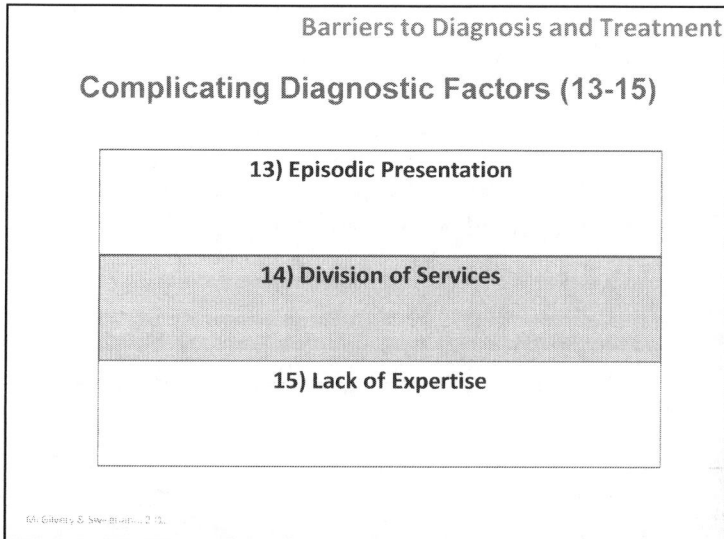

Barriers to Diagnosis and Treatment

Complicating Diagnostic Factors (13-15)

| 13) Episodic Presentation |
| 14) Division of Services |
| 15) Lack of Expertise |

13) Episodic Presentation –Significant mental health symptoms may come and go in an unpredictable manner. If a person is not displaying symptoms when he or she is assessed by a mental health professional, the presence of a mental health disorder may go undetected. As an example, an individual with bipolar disorder may be in a manic episode when an appointment is scheduled with his or her psychiatrist. By the time of the appointment, however, he or she may have cycled out of the manic episode and thus the symptoms of a mania may no longer be present when examined by the psychiatrist.

14) Division of Services –Even today, there exists a tendency for the administration and funding of mental health and intellectual/developmental disability services to be separate. Each system may expect the other to serve the individual who has a dual diagnosis. In addition, there may be a perception by staff in both types of systems that they are poorly equipped to provide appropriate services. Due to these factors, many individuals may be unable to access appropriate and comprehensive services.

15) Lack of Expertise –Typically, professionals receiving formal training in the realm of mental health (e.g., psychiatry, social work) receive minimal training regarding the issue of intellectual/developmental disability. Conversely, professionals trained to work with people with intellectual/developmental disability (e.g., psychologists, special education teachers) may receive extremely limited training in the realm of mental health disorders in persons with IDD. As a result, collaboration among professionals is required to ensure all significant issues in a person's life are understood and appropriately addressed.

MODULE II

Slide 56

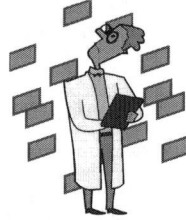

Psychiatric Symptoms/Learned Behaviors/Medication Conditions:

A Clinical Challenge

It can be difficult to distinguish whether a behavioral problem is associated with:

- **A symptom of a psychiatric disorder**
- **A learned behavior**
- **A medical condition**

Challenging behaviors, may at times, be related to the person's mental illness, while at other times they may be an expression of learned behavior. Often psychiatric symptoms and learned behaviors co-exist. Also, a medical condition can be a strong influence on challenging behavior. Mental illness and physical illness can both contribute to the function of behavior.

M
O
D
U
L
E

I
I

Slide 57

12 Indications that a Behavioral
Pattern may be the result of a
Psychiatric Condition

Slide 58

Assessment Considerations

Indications that a behavioral pattern may be the
result of a psychiatric condition

1. The behavior occurs in all environments; it is not
   just exhibited in specific settings

2. Behavioral strategies have been largely
   ineffective

3. The individual doesn't appear to have control
   over their behavior. He/she doesn't appear to be
   able to start or stop the behavior at will.

Adapted from Mapleton & Sweetland 2011

The following 4 slides present a list of different "tips" or "clues" that a behavior pattern may have a psychiatric origin. First, does the behavior occur in all settings? If the behavior does not seem to have any connection to the environment or features of the environment (school, home, and community; occurs with all different care providers and family), then the cause of the behavior might be internal. Second, have competent behavior intervention strategies been used with no effect. This is the most difficult one to judge, as simply having tried behavioral interventions may be meaningless if they were not well constructed. Third, does the person seem to make efforts to control the behavior with no success. Many patterns of behavior that do occur as a means for manipulating the environment or others do seem purposeful.

Slide 59

Assessment Considerations

Indications that a behavioral pattern may be the result of a psychiatric condition

4. There are changes in sleep patterns; increased, decreased or disturbed sleep.

5. The individual is experiencing excessive mood or unusual mood patterns.

6. There are changes in the individual's appearance and a decline in their independent living skills.

Adapted from *Aggression & Sweeney et al. 2001*

Significant change in sleep patterns may represent a sign of a psychiatric condition, though there are a legion of other causes, such as a side effect of a decongestant. When there is a change in behavior along with a change in sleep, that information may be of diagnostic use. Different types of psychiatric conditions may cause different disturbances in sleep. Changes in mood are a symptom of some kinds of psychiatric illness, and mood tracking may be suggested by clinical professionals. Changes in appearance and self care are of similar import. If somebody is normally quite fastidious, but suddenly stops bathing or combing one's hair, that may be an important bit of information.

Slide 60

Assessment Considerations

Indications that a behavioral pattern may be the
result of a psychiatric condition

7. The person may start to engage in purposeful self-
   harm (cutting, hitting, scratching, pulling out hair).

8. The person may start to show signs of
   hallucination, such as staring to the side or
   corners and not appear to track conversations.

9. There may be changes in eating patterns such as
   eating less or more.

Adapted from Megivern & Swanstrom, 2012

Items #7 and 8 are important and direct symptoms of some kinds of mental illness, and information about these should be immediately shared with clinical professionals. Chronic low level pulling out hair ("trichotillomania") may be more akin to a bad habit such as nail biting in some people, and is not a particularly significant warning sign in and of itself. Changes in eating, like changes in sleep(#4) should be monitored.

MODULE II

Slide 61

> ### Assessment Considerations
>
> Indications that a behavioral pattern may be the
> result of a psychiatric condition
>
> 10. The individual has a history of a psychiatric
> disorder that was in remission.
>
> 11. There is an acute onset of the behavior. If there is
> a particularly rapid onset with a significant change
> in mental status or cognitive functioning, rule out
> a possible delirium with an underlying medical
> cause.
>
> 12. There is an unusual change in behavior patterns,
> such as a significant change from baseline
> behavior
>
> Adapted from Mc|ennon & Sutherland, 20_2

#10 is very important, as psychiatric illness do go into and out of remission in some cases. Keeping a thorough record of prior psychiatric illness is necessary for this reason. If a person lives in a setting where staff turnover is frequent, prior knowledge of illness history can easily be forgotten. Good record keeping and review is important, as is knowledge of behavior patterns. Acute onset of changes in behavior are always of concern and should always be considered.

Slide 62

Medical Problems &
Problem Behavior

•Why do medical causes of problem behaviors get missed?

•Why do we have to be.......
    Sherlock Holmes?

Ask the participants to offer suggestions as to why medical problems are often missed in assessing behavior and mental health.

Slide 63

Medical Problems &
Problem Behavior

Medical conditions can be present when behavioral problems are exhibited.

Medication effects / reactions can be present when behavioral problems are exhibited.

Medical conditions are often underdiagnosed.

Medical conditions can mask as behavioral problems.

Medical conditions, including those associated with medications can be present when an individual with IDD exhibits a behavioral problem.

Limited verbal skills in persons with IDD complicate the diagnosing of comorbid medical problems. Frequently, the involved individual is not able to communicate his/her discomfort, distress, or pain.

Behaviors may be associated with a known health problem or a previously unrecognized health problem. General medical conditions of importance are pain or other discomfort, sleep disorders, atypical seizure disorders, and tic disorders, as well as problems associated with alcohol use, abuse, or abrupt withdrawal, and use of illegal drugs. Individuals with other health problems may have behavior problems associated with their general medical condition, such as behavior problems often seen with low blood sugar in people with diabetes and various behavioral symptoms associated with thyroid disease, both under-active and over-active thyroid or problems related to dental pain or discomfort expressed as behavioral symptoms.

Slide 64

Medical Problems & Problem Behavior

DRUG SIDE EFFECTS
Akathisia, Delirium, Dyskinesia
INFECTIONS
ENDOCRINOLOGICAL PROBLEMS
Thyroid problems   Diabetes
NEUROLOGICAL PROBLEMS
Epilepsy   Other movement problems
OTHER
Dental pain   Sleep apnea   Headaches
Hearing and vision problems   Back pain

People with IDD can experience a variety of medical conditions, and these medical conditions can influence the manifestation of behavioral problems.

There a number of medical conditions that can present as psychiatric symptoms or behavioral problems. It is therefore very important to assess medical conditions as part of the overall bio-psychosocial assessment. The following are some medical causes that can present as psychiatric symptoms:

- Endocrine disorders
- Nutritional deficiencies
- Neurological disorders
- Cardiovascular disorders
- Cancers
- Gastro-intestinal disorders
- Sensory disorders

Slide 65

Exercise

Each person to share information about a medication they know that has a relevant side effect.

Slide 66

Medical Problems & Problem Behavior

Medical Problems often under-recognized
Dental Problems often under-recognized

- **Medical/Dental problems can cause SIB**
- **Need to identify if there is an underlying physical problem**

Ruling out physical causes of challenging/problem behavior is a critical component of any biopsychosocial assessment, especially given the challenges a person with an IDD has in self-reporting pain or discomfort caused by an underlying medical or dental problem.

Slide 67

Medical Problems & Problem Behavior

Case Example of Dental Pain & SIB

- 28 year old female with IDD referred to dental office for routine exam
- Mother noted that she began pulling out her hair
- Dental exam showed a fractured upper molar tooth, & tooth was extracted
- Mother subsequently reported that hair pulling ceased

Slide 68

> Medical Problems &
> Problem Behavior
>
> ### Condensed Medical Data in Chart
>
> It is essential that all earlier medical data be available.
>
> It is important that the past and present medical history be condensed in a format that can be easily read and placed in the person's chart.

Medical information data gathering and placing it in the chart often occurs as a list of medical diagnoses in the past as well as all treatments for these conditions, usually in some sort of time-line form. While this list may take a great deal of time to develop and condense, this is usually time well spent.

A copy of the information should always be retained in files for whatever the current living situation may be, but should move with the individual. Copies can be provided to consultants as appropriate. Information should, of course, be updated frequently.

MODULE II

Slide 69

Medical conditions can, and often do, mask as mental health problems in people with IDD. This is a result of three variables :

• Medical problems are often not adequately diagnosed in persons with IDD.

• Limited communication skills make it difficult for the persons to express pain and discomfort.

• Third, typical signs and symptoms of a mental health disorder can reflect signs and symptoms of a medical condition.

Slide 70

The fact that medical conditions and mental illness look similar reinforces the need for an integrated model to ensure a comprehensive assessment and symptom tracking over time/settings to differentiate conditions.

For example, as indicated in this slide, symptoms of mania are the same as symptoms of Akathisia.

Symptoms of depression can be the same as symptoms of constipation.

Slide 71

Medical Problems & Problem Behavior

1. **Sleep Pattern**
   Quality and quantity of sleep can affect physical and mental health
   For example:
   a. Poor sleep ð fatigue ð irritability
   b. Depression ð poor sleep ð irritability
   c. Medical problem (discomfort caused by constipation) ð poor sleep ð irritability

   Assessment Strategy

   Maintain sleep data

The issue of poor sleep has the final pathway of resulting in irritability. It is important to assess the determinants that are causing the poor sleep and irritability. Is it a medical problem or is it a psychiatric problem? The answer to this question is based on collecting other information in addition to maintaining sleep data.

Slide 72

A change in appetite can be a clue to either a medical or psychiatric problem. The key to assessment of change in appetite is to monitor and document eating patterns and using this data along with other sources of information. This will help us to determine the primary cause of a change in food consumption.

Slide 73

MODULE II

A change in activity level, from baseline behavior, may be indicative of either a medical or psychiatric problem. It is, therefore, important to monitor and document changes in activity level as well as to monitor other signs and symptoms.

Slide 74

A person who has IDD, and has a declined activity level from baseline, may be exhibiting a medical problem or a psychiatric symptom. A change in one's level of activity, needs to be assessed from a holistic perspective.

The final pathway, in this example, non-compliant behavior, could be caused by either a medical problem or psychiatric condition.

Slide 75

> BEAMS
>
> - **Are there any changes in the current conditions?**
> - **Are there any changes in:**
>   - B = behavior
>   - E = energy level*
>   - A = appetite
>   - M = mood
>   - S = sleep patterns
> - **How long the symptoms/changes have been occurring?**
> - **Is there anything that appears to help the person feel better when these signs are present?**
> - **In what context have these changes occurred?**

The BEAMS assessment can act as a pre-screening for mental illness. Direct support professionals can collect data on observations of changes in current conditions to mental health/health professionals to help direct assessment for medical/mental health issues.

* While previous slides refer to change of activity level as an indicator, energy level is used in this tool but can be used in the same manner as activity level although it does include factors such as lethargy and hyperactivity.

M
O
D
U
L
E

I
I

References: Module II

Baer, D.M., Wolf, M.M., & Risley, T.R. (1968). Some current dimensions of applied behavior analysis. *Journal of Applied Behavior Analysis, 1*(1), 91–97.

Beasley, J.B., Kroll, J., & Sovner, R. (1992). Community-based crisis mental health services for persons with developmental disabilities: The START model. *The Habilitative Mental Healthcare Newsletter, 11* (9), 55-57.

Beavers, G.A., Iwata, B.A., & Lerman, D.C. (2013). Thirty years of research on the functional analysis of problem behavior. *Journal of Applied Behavior Analysis, 46*(1), 1-21.

Carr, J.E, & Sidener, T.M. (2002). On the relation between applied behavior analysis and positive behavioral support. *The Behavior Analyst, 25*, 245–253.

Charlot, L., Abend, S., Ravin, P., Mastis, K., Hunt, A., & Deutsch, C., (2011). Non-psychiatric health problems among psychiatric inpatients with intellectual disabilities. *Journal of Intellectual Disability Research, 5, 199-209.*

Engel, G. (1977). The need for a new medical model: a challenge for biomedicine. *Science. 196*(4286), 129-196.

Griffiths, D. & Gardner, W. (2002). The integrated biopsychosocial approach to challenging behaviours. In Griffiths, D., Stavrakaki, C., & Summers, J. (Eds.). *Dual diagnosis: An introduction to the mental health needs of persons with developmental disabilities.* Sudbury, ON: Habilitative Mental Health Resource Network.

Hawkins, B. (1999). Rights, place of residence and retirement: Lessons from case studies on aging. In S. Herr, & G. Weber (Eds.), *Aging, rights and quality of life* Baltimore, MD: Brookes.

Haveman, M.J., Heller, T., Lee, L.A, Maaskant, M.A, Shooshtari, S., & Strydom, A. (2009). Report on the State of Science on Health Risks and Ageing in People with Intellectual Disabilities. IASSID Special Interest Research Group on Ageing and Intellectual Disabilities/Faculty Rehabilitation Sciences, University of Dortmund.

Iwata, B.A., Dorsey, M.F., Slifer, K.J., Bauman, K.E., & Richman, G.S.(1994). Toward a functional analysis of self-injury. *Journal of Applied Behavioral Analysis, 27*(2), 197-209.

McClinock, K., Hall, S. & Oliver, C.(2003). Risk markers associated with challenging behaviours in people with developmental disabilities: a meta-analytic study. *Journal of Intellectual Disability Research, 47*, 40-416.

McGilvery, S., & Sweetland, D. (2011). *Intellectual disability and mental health: A training manual in dual diagnosis.* Kingston, NY: NADD Press.

Morrison, A.K., & Gillig, P.M. (2012). Psychiatric assessment. In J.P. Gentile. & P.M. Gillig, (Eds.), *Psychiatry of intellectual disability: A practical manual* (pp. 14-25). Oxford, UK: John Wiley & Sons, Ltd.

Poindexter, A. R. (2005). *Assessing medical issues associated with behavioural/ psychiatric problems in persons with intellectual disability.* Kingston, NY: NADD Press.

Reiss, S., Leviton, G.W., & Szyszko, J. (1982). Emotional disturbance and mental retardation: diagnostic overshadowing. *American Journal of Mental Deficiency, 86*(6), 567-574.

Sovner, R., & Hurley, A. D. (1989). Ten diagnostic principles for recognizing psychiatric disorder in mentally retarded persons. *Psychiatric Aspects of Mental Retardation Reviews. 8,* 9-14.

MODULE II

M
O
D
U
L
E

I
I

Mental Health Evaluations

Slide 1

Module III

Mental Health Evaluation:
Mental Status Examinations
(MSE)

Slide 2

This module includes information about best practices in mental health evaluation for persons with IDD with a focus on mental status examination (MSE).

MODULE III

Slide 3

Learning Objectives

- Summarize the importance of assessing the cognitive developmental level of the person with IDD as it pertains to Mental Status Examination
- Describe three components of the Mental Status Examination
- Describe the 11 domains and how they are pertinent to the assessment process
- Describe how the developmental level of the person is related to the assessment process
- Articulate the purpose of the DSM and how it is used in the diagnostic process

Slide 4

Definitions

Affect: the observable expression of emotion

Psychomotor activity: movement or muscle activity related to mental processes

Thought process: brain processing information to form concepts, make decisions, reason, and problem solve

Cognitive functions: the mental processes involved in gaining knowledge and comprehension - thinking, knowing, remembering, judging, and problem-solving. These are higher-level functions of the brain and encompass language, imagination, perception, and planning.

Judgement: process by which people make decisions and form conclusions based on available information and material combined with thought and experience

Insight: self-understanding – the awareness of own attitudes, feelings, and behavior

Slide 5

Effects of IDD in Clinical Presentation

The interaction between IDD and MI are a result of four factors that reflect the profound biopsychosocial affects of developmental disabilities

1. Intellectual Distortion

2. Psychosocial Masking

3. Cognitive Disintegration

4. Baseline Exaggeration

All four of these factors are critical to examine in the clinical presentation of a person with IDD who also has MI. Part of the traditional difficulty in proper diagnosis in this population comes from these four concerns. Each will be discussed in turn.

Slide 6

Four Nonspecific Factors Associated with IDD That Influence the Diagnostic Process

Factor 1: Intellectual Distortion

Definition: Refers to the developmental effects of IDD on the person's diminished ability to think abstractly and communicate intelligibly

Clinical Impact: Inability for person to label his/her own experiences and report them

Example: When asked if he/she "hears voices", the person might respond "yes" without fully comprehending the implication of the question

MODULE III

In the general population, diagnosis of an MI often is made based on an interview of the person with a standard set of questions. A person with IDD may not have the intellectual function to understand the question, communicate about experiences, remember experiences, or have the self awareness to reflect on changes in perception or what is "normal." One of the common interview questions is about hearing voices. What might happen if a person answers "yes" because he or she hears the interviewer asking the question?

Slide 7

> **Mental Health Evaluation**
>
> Four Nonspecific Factors Associated with IDD That Influence the Diagnostic Process
>
> **Factor 2: Psychosocial Masking**
>
> <u>Definition</u>: Impoverished social skills and life experiences can influence the content of psychiatric symptoms
>
> <u>Clinical Impact</u>: The person with IDD might present significant symptomology that occurs within the developmental framework
>
> <u>Example</u>: A person with moderate level of IDD, might believe he/she can drive a car and this can be a manifestation of grandiosity
>
> Source: 1986

This refers to differences in the psychosocial lives of persons with IDD masking the presence of an MI. The lives of people with IDD often are very different from those of neurotypical people. Knowledge of the lives of people with IDD is crucial in understanding enough to make a competent diagnosis.

Slide 8

Mental Health Evaluation

Four Nonspecific Factors Associated with IDD That Influence the Diagnostic Process

Factor 3: Cognitive Disintegration

Definition: Stress-induced disruption of information processing – Tendency of person with IDD to become disorganized under stress

Clinical Impact: Bizarre presentation and psychotic-like state may be misdiagnosed as schizophrenia

Example: Vulnerability to high levels of stress and overload of cognitive functioning may lead to atypical clinical presentation

---

While it is true that many people under stress experience some degree of cognitive disintegration, due to the overall difficulties in cognition and typically less developed stress management skills, this is a more significant problem for people with IDD. Cognitive disintegration has resulted in many mis-diagnoses. Pressurized speech can occur under conditions of stress, but it is also a symptom of Schizophrenia, and in our clinical experience, people with IDD have ended up on neuroleptics as a result.

Slide 9

> **Mental Health Evaluation**
>
> Four Nonspecific Factors Associated with IDD That Influence the Diagnostic Process
>
> **Factor 4: Baseline Exaggeration**
>
> **Definition:** Pre-existing maladaptive behaviors, that were not attributed to mental illness, may increase in frequency and intensity with the onset of a psychiatric disorder
>
> **Clinical Impact:** Creates difficulty in establishing illness features, target symptoms, and outcome measures
>
> **Example:** SIB (Self Injurious Behavior) or aggression, that occurred infrequently may suddenly increase in severity at onset of a psychiatric disorder

Baseline exaggeration can be a significant problem with making a good diagnosis, as the frequency of problem behavior may go up, and then care providers only see the escalating problem behavior and only want to respond to that, rather than paying attention to other symptoms which also may be occurring.

Slide 10

> **The Mental Status Exam**
>
> • The Mental Status Exam can only be administered by a regulated health or mental health professional such as a physician, nurse, psychologist or psychiatrist.   **CAUTION**
>
> •A direct support professional can contribute to the process by being familiar with the components of the exam and the information they may need to assist the person to receive an accurate assessment.

M O D U L E   I I I

The mental status examination is intended to be one part of a comprehensive assessment of a person's overall condition. It is infrequent that this process would be completed by physician or nurse but they are qualified to administer it. More frequently, this will be completed by a mental health professional: psychologist or psychiatrist.

It is outside the scope of practice for a direct support professional from any discipline to conduct this examination. However, it is important to be familiar with the components of the exam to be able to provide thoughtful and informed contributions, if needed, to the assessment process. A direct support professional needs to be prepared to provide a comprehensive history of the person, his or her medical conditions, normative behavior/baseline behavior, and any previous assessment results including results of functional assessment/ analysis of behavior. The clinician will need to understand the nature of a presenting problem, who defined it and how, the history of the problem, how long it has been observed, in what environments it is observed, if it is long standing, and why assessment is being sought. (Fletcher, Loschen, Stavrakaki, & First, 2007)

Slide 11

> **Mental Status Examination (MSE)**
>
> - Systemic observation and recording about a person's thinking, emotions, and behavior
> - **MSE for people with IDD needs to be modified**
> - Useful way to organize and standardize the data of patient observation
> - **MSE is a snapshot of the mental status at the time of the assessment. The MSE can be used as a tool to note change in the status from one point-in-time to another.**
> - MSE is a diagnostic measurement. Data from care providers and patient history can be helpful.

Along with other components such as the history of the presenting complaint, family history, current and past medical history, the mental status examination can provide more detailed information to formulate a psychiatric diagnosis and to direct any further assessments which need to take place: adaptive functioning assessment, cognitive assessments, psychometric testing, etc.

Slide 12

```
Mental Status Examination (MSE)

  I.   General Appearance & Behavior
  II.  Mood and Affect
  III. Psychomotor Activity and Speech
  IV.  Thought Process and Content
  V.   Cognitive Function
  VI.  Judgment and Insight

Levitas, Hurley & Pary, 2001
```

The purpose of a Mental Status Exam (MSE) is to get a comprehensive cross-section of the person's mental state.

An MSE is essentially the equivalent of a physical health exam but focuses on the behaviors and the mental state of the patient as opposed to the physical health. It provides a quick snapshot of the mental state at the time of the assessment and can be used as a tool to note change in status from one point in time to another.

The MSE records both the clinician's observation of the person's mental and emotional functioning at the time of assessment and responses to specific questions. The direct support professional's input may be required for the observational process as well as the interview process when the person being assessed has an intellectual/developmental disability. Contributions would be needed to assist the clinician to understand what baseline behavior looks like for the person, i.e., what the person's behaviors are like in general as they may appear quite different from those of a person who does not have an intellectual/developmental disability. Assistance may also be needed during the question/answer portion of the assessment for any number of reasons that are explicated further in this section.

Slide 13

> **Mental Status Examination (MSE)**
>
> I. **General Appearance & Behavior**
> - **Assesses person's attentiveness and effective participation in interview**
> - **Notes persons attitude toward examiner**
> - **Assesses posture and general motor activity**
> - **Notes facial expression**
> - **Notes personal hygiene and grooming**
> - **Assesses weight status**
>
> Levitas, Hurley & Pary, 2001
>
> **Note : All of the above is based on the cognitive developmental level of the individual with IDD.**

- Level of consciousness: if person is awake, alert, or sedated
- Participation in interview: the person with IDD may have significant limitations with regard to his/her participation in the interview. This is associated with limitations in expressive and receptive language skills.
- Attitude toward examiner: e.g., cooperative, guarded, suspicious
- Posture and general motor activity : e.g., rigid, tense, restless, pacing
- Facial expression: e.g., tearful, laughing, smiling, angry
- Personal hygiene and grooming : e.g., unkempt appearance, meticulous grooming
- Weight status: e.g., obesity, extreme thinness

MODULE III

Slide 14

> ### Mental Status Examination (MSE)
>
> I. General Appearance & Behavior (cont.)
> - The clinician may need to rely on collateral information about the person's baseline appearance and behavior
> - Baseline for a person with IDD may be very different from the neuro-typical person. For example, in a person with ASD, body posturing, self-hugging, and finger flicking may be the typical baseline behavior for a person on the Spectrum
>
> **Note : All of the above is based on the cognitive developmental level of the individual with IDD.**

For a person with an IDD, direct support professionals may be needed to provide baseline information on all the above observations so the assessor has information on what the person's general appearance and behavior are like. Baseline appearance and behavior can differ significantly from that of the general population. For example, for a person with ASD, the examiner may note the person's lack of eye contact. However, lack of eye contact is relatively "typical" for a person with ASD so this behavior is baseline for them. Similarly, body posturing, self-hugging, finger-flicking, and other behavior may be "typical" for the person, but be interpreted differently if the assessor does not have information about what is general behavior for the person.

Slide 15

> # Exercise
>
> **Appearance in relation to …….**
> **Body Build …..**
> **Clothing Appropriate to…**
> **Clean, neat, tidy, …..**
> **Hygiene and grooming ….**
> **Odor …**
> **Facial expression ….**
> **Eye Contact ….**
> **Other things that are noteworthy……**

Have the participants list examples of possible observations on appearance and behavior. Ask the participants to think of various people with IDD they have known and generate things that might have been observed about them for each question.

Slide 16

> **Mental Status Examination (MSE)**
>
> **II. Mood and Affect**
>
> - **Describe predominant mood**
> - **Describe affect including range**
>
> Note : All of the above is based on the cognitive developmental level of the individual with IDD.

MODULE III

- Describe predominant mood, e.g., neutral, anxious, fearful, elated, euphoric, depressed, angry, irritable

- Describe affect including range (e.g., broad, restricted, labile or changes easily); intensity (e.g., blunted, flat, animated); and appropriateness of mood/thought content

Once again, the direct support professional will need to assist the assessor to understand what typical mood and behavior are for the person and to interpret affect through behavioral expression.

Slide 17

Affect, in this context, refers to the observable expression of emotion. Given that many people who have intellectual disability have an affect that can be considered inconsistent with their emotional state, it is critical that the direct support professional provide the assessor with information on the general affect of the person.

For example, a person who has Cornelia de Lange Syndrome has difficulty with the facial expression of emotion. In absence of this information, an assessor could inappropriately interpret that the person has a flat affect, when this is the person's typical expression of emotion. Observation of behavior carries more import in this person's case than for someone in the general population.

Slide 18

> # Exercise
>
> ## II. Mood and affect
>
> - Appropriateness of affect /Appropriate or inappropriate to situation. Congruous / Incongruous
> - Range of affect …
> - Stability of affect ….
> - Attitude during encounter ….
> - Specific mood or feelings ….observed or reported
> - Anxiety Level Rate …..

Have the participants list examples of possible observations on appearance and behavior.

Slide 19

> **Mental Status Examination (MSE)**
>
> ### III. Psychomotor Activity and Speech
>
> - Assesses psychomotor activity and notes
>   - Rate of psychomotor activity (e.g., agitated, slowed)
>   - Presence of abnormal movements
> - Assesses speech and notes amount, volume, rate, organization of speech
>
> **Note : All of the above is based on the cognitive developmental level of the individual with IDD.**

- Assesses psychomotor activity and notes

- Rate of psychomotor activity (e.g., agitated, retarded)
- Presence of abnormal movements (grimacing, mannerisms, stereotype)
- Assesses speech and notes amount, volume, rate, organization of speech

Slide 20

> **Mental Status Examination (MSE)**
>
> **III. Psychomotor Activity and Speech (cont.)**
>
> - **Examiner will need other collateral data in understanding the typical psychomotor activity and speech organization for the person.**
>   - **For example, people who have Fragile X often have difficulty with gross motor coordination, which may lead to assessment as abnormal movements in absence of information about the effect of the syndrome.**
>
> **Note : All of the above is based on the cognitive developmental level of the individual with IDD.**
>
> Levitas, Hurley & Pary, 2001

As with previous sections of the examination, the direct support professional will need to assist the assessor in understanding the typical psychomotor activity and speech organization for the person. Many people who have IDD also have challenges with hyperactivity, challenges with gait, challenges with coordination, and challenges with verbal communication.

For examle, a person with William Syndrome frequently experiences emotional immaturity exhibited by over-reaction to events and exaggerated displays of fear, excitement, sadness, happiness, etc.

Slide 21

Exercise

III. Psychomotor Behavior
- Gait ...
- Handshake ...
- Abnormal movements ...
- Posture ....
- Rate of movements ...
- Co-ordination of

Have the participants list examples of possible observations on psychomotor behavior.

Slide 22

Mental Status Examination (MSE)

IV. Thought Process and Content
- Assess thought abnormalities
- Evaluate the content of thought
- Notes presence of delusions/ hallucinations (if so, what type of hallucinations)

Note : All of the above is based on the cognitive developmental level of the individual with IDD.

Rich fantasy life and self-talk are frequently associated with many types of IDD, especially Down syndrome. There is an extensive clinical history of this being in-

MODULE III

terpreted as delusional behavior leading to misdiagnosis of schizophrenia. In the absence of the knowledge that these traits are "typical" for a person with Down syndrome and the ability to accurately describe their context, assessment on a Mental Status Exam could conclude that these behaviors are abnormal.

Slide 23

Mental Status Examination (MSE)

IV. Thought Process and Content (cont.)

- **Clinical challenge in identifying abnormal thoughts and perceptions related to mental illness, compared to behaviors associated with the cognitive / developmental level of the individual**

- **Similarities between behaviors normal in young children without IDD and adults with IDD (i.e., self talk, imaginary friends, and rich fantasy life)**

Note : All of the above is based on the cognitive developmental level of the individual with IDD.

Levitas, Hurley & Pary, 2001

Assess thought abnormalities in logic, organization of words and phrases, association of ideas, and comprehensibility

Evaluate the content of thought, noting presence of ideas of reference, paranoid ideation, delusions (if so, what type of delusions), obsessions, compulsions, and phobias. Inquire about suicidal/homicidal ideation. People who have an IDD, particularly those in the moderate to profound ranges, may have difficulty accurately describing thoughts and feelings. In the more severe and profound ranges, they will likely have few verbal communication skills. Lack of meaningful communication complicates assessment of thought processes and content and the presence of delusions and hallucinations. Careful observation of behavior is critical for accurate assessment. The direct support professional will be relied upon to assist in observing and interpreting behavior.

Note presence of delusions, hallucinations if any. It is extremely difficult, if not impossible, to identify the existence of hallucinations and delusions in persons who have significant impairments in verbal communication. People with mild/

moderate levels of IDD can usually express their internal thought process. However, people at the lower end of the IDD range may not be able to communicate their internal states.

Delusions involve false beliefs relating to misinterpretations of perceptions and experiences despite evidence to the contrary. For example, someone may believe they are being followed or "spied on" by interpreting gestures, movements, song lyrics, newspaper articles, etc., as related to them when they are not.

Hallucinations involves perceiving things that aren't really there, i.e., the mind is responding to sensory stimuli that do not exist outside of the mind. An example of a hallucination is a feeling that bugs are crawling on one's skin when, in fact, there are none.

Slide 24

Exercise

I. Thought Process
Clarity
Relevance / logic
Flow
Rapidly shifting ideas/thoughts?...
Perseveration ...
Pressure of speech ....
II. Content
Thoughts content consistent with reality?

Levitas Hurley & Fary, 2001.

Have the participants list examples of possible observations on thought process and content.

Slide 25

Mental Status Examination (MSE)

V. Cognitive Function

- Assess orientations to time, place, and persons
- Evaluate attention and concentration
- Assess memory
- Assess intellectual functioning

Note : All of the above is based on the cognitive developmental level of the individual with IDD.

Assess person's orientations to time, place and persons. Note: A person with IDD may not know how to tell time, but this does not mean that there is a cognitive deficit relative to the person's level of IQ with regard to an MSE. A person with IDD should be able to tell you what city he or she lives in, but not necessarily the street address, and this should be considered normative, given the person's developmental level.

Evaluate person's attention and concentration. Note: Attention and concentration should be evaluated with consideration of the person's developmental level.

Assess person's memory. Note: Detailed information and chronology of events in the past need to be considered relative to the person's developmental age.

Note: The examiner will need to assess intellectual functioning based on estimating the person's level of functioning. For example a person with an IQ of 68 is below normative range of intellectual functioning. However, an IQ of 68 is at the high end of mild level of intellectual/developmental disability.

Slide 26

Mental Status Examination (MSE)

V. Cognitive Function (cont.)

- Detailed information and chronology of events need to be considered relative to the person's developmental age. For example, they may remember the names of their siblings and which are older and younger; but may not be able to remember the exact age of each sibling.

- The examiner will need to assess intellectual functioning based on estimating the person's level of functioning.

Note : All of the above is based on the cognitive developmental level of the individual with IDD.

A person with IDD may remember events that have importance to them. For example, they may remember that we eat turkey during Thanksgiving. Another example is they may remember the names of their siblings and which are older and younger; but may not be able to remember the exact age of each sibling.

Assess intellectual functioning.

MODULE III

Slide 27

Exercise

V. Cognitive Function

- Attention & Concentration ….
- Memory….
- Abstraction Concrete thinking…..
- Orientation ….

Have the participants list examples of possible observations on cognitive functioning

Slide 28

Mental Status Examination (MSE)

VI. Judgment and Insight

- Assess judgment in general

- Evaluates insight in situation and illness

> Note : All of the above is based on the cognitive developmental level of the individual with IDD.

Judgment and insight need to be based on the person's developmental level.

The clinician needs to keep in mind a developmental perspective when assessing judgment and insight with regard to a person with IDD.

For example, a 16 year old adolescent with moderate level of IDD (IQ of 35-55) would not be expected to have a great deal of abilities regarding judgment and would have limited if any insight as to the nature of the problem for which he/she was brought to the clinician's attention.

Slide 29

> # Exercise
>
> **VI. Judgement and Insight ....**
>
> **Impulsive behavior ....**
> **Insight into illness ....**
> **Examples....**
>
> L. allan, Huntley & Hary, 2001

Have the participants list examples of possible observations on judgement and insight.

References Module III

Fletcher, R., Loschen, E., Stavrakaki, C., & First, M. (2007) *Diagnostic manual-Intellecual disability (DM-ID): A textbook of diagnosis of mental disorders in persons with intellectual disability.* Kingston, NY: NADD Press.

Levitas, A.S., Hurley, A.D., & Pary, R. (2001). The mental status examination in patients with mental retardation and developmental disabilities. *Mental Health Aspects of Developmental Disabilities, 4*(1), 1-16.

Sovner, R. (1986). Limiting factors in the use of DSM-III criteria with mentally ill/mentally retarded persons. *Psychopharmacology Bulletin, 22,* 1055-1059.

M
O
D
U
L
E

I
I
I

Signs and Symptoms of Mental Illness

Slide 1

> # Module IV
>
> ## Signs and Symptoms of Mental Illness

Slide 2

> This module includes information regarding Signs and Symptoms of Depressive Disorders, Bipolar Disorder, Anxiety Disorders, Personality Disorders, and Psychosis.
>
> The module highlights the importance of observation and behavioral equivalence.

Slide 3

Learning Objectives

- List three signs commonly present in people who have ID and the following diagnoses:
  - Depression
  - Bipolar Disorder
  - Anxiety
  - Personality Disorders
  - Psychosis
- Articulate the importance of observation in the assessment process.

Slide 4

DEPRESSION

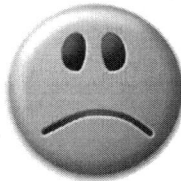

Slide 5

> Depression
>
> The prevalence of depression among adults with intellectual/developmental disability is estimated to be 2.2%.
>
> Deb, Thomas, and Bright, 2001

Slide 6

> Depression
>
> - **Can significantly disrupt school, work, family relationships, social life, etc.**
>
> - **Onset tends to be more insidious and changes less dramatic** (Deb et al., 2001)
>
> - **Increased prevalence in some symptoms as compared to typical population** (Matson et al., 1988)
>
> - **Depression is among the most common psychiatric disorders in persons with IDD** (Lamon & Reiss, 1987)
>
> Hughes, 2005

Depression is characterized by low mood, accompanied by slowing of thinking and difficulty concentrating and sustaining energy. There is change of appetite, poor sleep, typically early morning wakening, and physical movement may be slowed. There is little doubt that depressive illness occurs even in individuals

M
O
D
U
L
E

I
V

with severe intellectual disability, and it is likely that this is significantly underdiagnosed. This is not surprising, as the individual has reduced ability to disclose or describe his or her mood, and the psychiatrist is thereby denied access to the cardinal symptoms of affective illness.

Slide 7

Depression

Public Figures who have/had Depression

- Abraham Lincoln, U.S. President
- Isaac Newton, Scientist
- Buzz Aldrin, Astronaut
- Terry Bradshaw, Former Quarterback
- Drew Carey, Actor/Comedian
- Leo Tolstoy, Author

Slide 8

DSM 5 Symptom for Depression	Presentation in Someone with IDD
DSM-5: Change in terminology to Major Depressive Disorder	•Frequent unexplained crying •Decrease in laughter and smiling •General irritability and subsequent aggression or self-injury •Sad facial expression
Markedly diminished interest or pleasure in all, or almost all, activities most of the day nearly every day	•No longer participates in favorite activities •Reinforcers no longer valued •Increased time spent alone •Refusals of most work/social activities

Depression

The DSM criteria subsets are listed on the left side. The right side lists the manifestations in a person with IDD. The right side is a listing of behavioral observations or behavioral equivalents to what is listed in the criteria subsets of the DSM.

Note the importance of observation over time for accurate diagnosis of any psychiatric illness.

Depressed mood can be observed, e.g., sad facial expression or crying.

A loss of interest in pleasurable activities can be observed, i.e., the person no longer attending the activities from which he/she derived pleasure.

MODULE IV

Slide 9

DSM 5 Symptom for Depression	Presentation in Someone with IDD
Weight Change/ Appetite Change	•Measured weight changes •Increased refusals to come to table to eat •Unusually disruptive at meal times •Constant food seeking behaviors
Insomnia	•Disruptive at bed time •Repeatedly gets up at night •Difficulty falling asleep •No longer gets up for work/activities •Early morning awakening
Hypersomnia	•Over 12 hours of sleep per day •Naps frequently

Depression

Through either self report for people with mild levels of IDD or through obtaining data from informants we can identify if there are any changes in weight and sleep patterns. A change in weight or sleep patterns can be a clear indication of depression.

Slide 10

DSM 5 Symptom for Depression	Presentation in Someone with IDD
Psychomotor Agitation	•Restless, Fidgety, Pacing •Increased disruptive behavior
Psychomotor Retardation	•Sits for extended periods •Moves slowly •Takes longer than usual to complete activities

Depression

It is sometimes possible to elicit from others a history of recent psychomotor retardation or psychomotor agitation. Psychomotor agitation can be observed when the person is irritated/restless. On the other hand psychomotor retardation can be observed when the person's motor activity seems to be slower than baseline behavior. Baseline behavior is the "typical" behavior the person displays before any intervention is started; in other words, behavior that is steady in form, frequency, and intensity even before any treatment or intervention is started.

Slide 11

	Depression
DSM 5 Symptom for Depression	**Presentation in Someone with IDD**
Fatigue/Loss of Energy	●Needs frequent breaks to complete simple activity ●Slumped/tired body posture ●Does not complete tasks with multiple steps
Inappropriate guilt	●Statements like "I'm dumb," "I'm retarded," etc. ●Seeming to seek punishment ●Social isolation

Hughes, 2010

A person with IDD can express fatigue/loss of energy through difficulty in completing tasks, and the fatigue or loss of energy can be observed through body posture.

Feelings of worthlessness can be difficult to elicit in a person with limited verbal skills. However, those with mild/moderate levels of IDD will often make self-deprecating statements such as "I'm stupid."

MODULE IV

Slide 12

DSM 5 Symptom for Depression	Presentation in Someone with IDD
Lack of Concentration/ Diminished Ability to Think/Indecisiveness	•Decreased work output •Does not stay with tasks •Decrease in IQ upon retesting
Thoughts of Death	•Preoccupation with family member's death •Talking about committing or attempting suicide •Fascination with violent movies/television shows

Depression

Lack of concentration can be observed by one's inability to stay on task and maintain focus.

Thoughts of death are difficult to observe in a person with severe/profound levels of IDD. However, a person with some level of verbal skills may, for example, have a pre-occupation with themes of death and dying.

Please note: The lists of symptoms are intended to be representative of the most common symptoms for Depression. These lists are not intended to be exhaustive or reflective of symptoms of other Mood Disorders.

Slide 13

Depression, like other disorders, should be treated using a multi-modal approach. A comprehensive treatment plan should include a multi-disciplinary approach. No single approach should be used alone. For example, short term medication treatment combined with other habilitative approaches should be the protocol embraced.

MODULE IV

Slide 14

What symptoms of depression might look like for a person with IDD…

Set Up:	Set Off:	So I:	And I get or avoid:
Depression Not that interested in work.	Cued regarding going to work	Ignore the cue and become aggressive	Avoid going to work. Work and paycheck used to be an incentive, but due to depression, formerly preferred events are no longer preferred.

Ask the group to think of another example following the set up above.

Slide 15

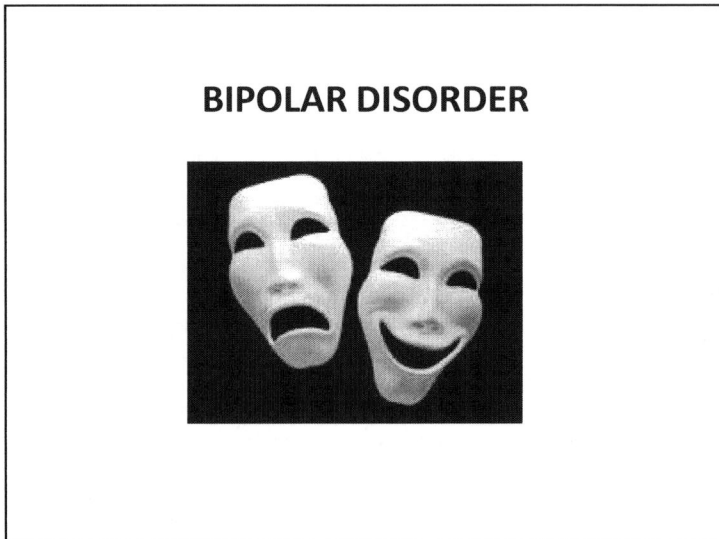

BIPOLAR DISORDER

Slide 16

Bipolar Disorder

- **Causes mood swings**

- Persons with Bipolar Disorder may have periods of mania and periods of depression as well as normal moods.

- The length of cycle between moods can vary between rapid cycling or more slowly over time.

- **Only a minority of people alternate back and forth between mania and depression with each cycle; in most, one or the other predominates to some extent. (Beers & Berkow, 1999)**

- During a manic episode, a person will display oversupply of confidence and energy

Beers & Berkow, 1999

Bipolar Disorder is an illness that causes extreme mood swings. A person with Bipolar Disorder may have periods of mania, periods of depression, and periods of normal moods. During an episode of mania, an individual will typically have an oversupply of confidence and energy that may lead to reckless or dangerous behavior. The length of a manic or depressed cycle may last from days to months. Without treatment, Bipolar Disorder can lead to poor job performance, financial difficulties, problems with family and friends, and death from reckless behavior or suicide.

MODULE IV

Slide 17

Public Figures who have/had Bipolar Disorder

- Carrie Fisher, Actor/Author
- Linda Hamilton, Actor
- Catherine Zeta Jones, Actor
- Vincent Van Gogh, Artist (suspected)
- Jane Pauley, Journalist
- Sting, Musician
- Ludwig van Beethoven, Composer/Musician (suspected)

Slide 18

Bipolar Disorder

DSM 5 Symptoms of Mania	Presentation in Someone with IDD
Elevated, expansive, or irritable mood and abnormally and persistently increasing goal-directed activity or energy	• Smiling, hugging or being affectionate with people who previously were not favored by the individual • **Boisterousness** • **Over-reactivity to small incidents** • **Extreme excitement** • **Excessive laughing and giggling** • **Self-injury associated with irritability** • **Enthusiastic greeting of everyone**

Hughes 2000.

The manifestation of euphoric, elevated or irritable mood in a person with IDD can be observed. Episodic motor over-activity and extreme excitement are common symptoms among people with IDD.

Slide 19

DSM 5 Symptoms of Mania	Presentation in Someone with IDD
Increased energy or activity and 3 or more of the following: Inflated self-esteem/grandiosity Decreased need for sleep More talkative/pressured speech Flight of ideas Distractibility Increase in psychomotor agitation Excessive involvement in activities that have a high potential for painful consequences	• Behavioral challenges when prompted to go to try to sleep • Constantly getting up at night • Seems rested after not sleeping (i.e., not irritable due to lack of sleep as is common in depression)

Bipolar Disorder

People in a manic phase generally have decreased need for sleep. This can be disruptive to others as the manic person may be pacing while others are trying to sleep. Lack of sleep related to mania is a physiological symptom and accommodations need to be made for it as a result.

Slide 20

DSM 5 Symptoms of Mania	Presentation in Someone with IDD
Inflated Self-esteem/ Grandiosity	• Making improbable claims (e.g., is a staff member, has mastered all necessary skills, etc.) • Dramatic physical presentation • Dressing provocatively • Demanding rewards
Flight of Ideas	• Disorganized speech • Thoughts not connected • Quickly changing subjects

Bipolar Disorder

Inflated self esteem/grandiosity: for example, a person with IDD might make claims of having the ability to drive a car or having a profession that is well beyond his or her ability.

Flights of ideas are difficult to ascertain in a person with no verbal skills. However in a person with mild/moderate levels of IDD, a disorganization of speech can occur in a manic stage.

Slide 21

DSM 5 Symptoms of Mania	Presentation in Someone with IDD
More Talkative/ Pressured Speech	• Increased singing • Increased swearing • Perseverative speech • Screaming • Frequent interrupting • Non-verbal communication increases • Increase in vocalizations

Bipolar Disorder

Hughes, 2016

The presentation of pressured speech in a person with mild/moderate levels of IDD is similar to individuals who do not have IDD.

For people at the severe/profound level of IDD, the presentation of pressured speech may be screaming or an increase in volume, pressure, or repetitiveness of the way the person communicates. For example, an increase in grunting sounds.

Slide 22

DSM 5 Symptoms of Mania	Presentation in Someone with IDD
Distractibility	• Decrease in work/task performance • Leaving tasks incomplete • Inability to settle (e.g., stay seated and focus on favorite TV show, stay seated through a complete activity when generally able to do so)

Bipolar Disorder

The presentation of distractibility can be observed in a person with IDD. The individual shows reduced productivity at work or day program. When he or she is asked to do activities that require concentration, he or she may have unexplained "skill loss" or may be unable to finish their tasks.

Slide 23

Bipolar Disorder

DSM 5 Symptoms of Mania	Presentation in Someone with IDD
Agitation/Increase in Goal Directed Behavior	• Pacing • Negativism • Working on many activities at once • Fidgeting • Aggression • Rarely sits
Excessive Pleasurable Activities	• Increase in masturbation • Giving away/spending money

MODULE IV

Observers may report that the individual with IDD engages in activities in a "sped up manner," rarely sits down, paces, and walks rapidly.

Excessive pleasurable activities may include the individual with IDD engaging in more sexual behavior or talk, reporting more sexual activity, or masturbating frequently, increased eating, etc. Symptoms would be more apparent/disruptive in a shared living environment.

Negativism, in this context, refers to resisting suggestions, advice or direction. It is a behavioral attitude common in a variety of disorders including Bipolar Disorder.

Please note: The lists of symptoms are intended to be representative of the most common symptoms for Bipolar Disorder. These lists are not intended to be exhaustive or reflective of symptoms of other Mood Disorders.

Slide 24

Bipolar Disorder

Treatment Strategies

- **Psychotherapy with a focus on understanding and managing the disorder**

- Environmental and social modification (i.e., increase supervision to ensure safety)

- **Positive support strategies**

- Mood stabilizing and antidepressant medication

A treatment approach needs to be multi-faceted and multi-disciplinary. The first line of treatment is likely to be medication treatment. This is to assist the individual to become more stable in order to benefit from other treatment and habilitative approaches. Once the person is stabilized then other supports can come into play, such as psychotherapy and positive support strategies, focus on wellness and other supports as needed.

Slide 25

What symptoms of bi-polar disorder might look like for a person with IDD...

Set Up:	Set Off:	So I:	And I get or avoid:
Bi-polar cycling into manic phase Not always a good sleeper Not a lot of friends	Want to continue activity for many hours into the night Staff interrupt the activity	I begin to scream and wake up the rest of the house	Staff allow me to return to activity since it is quieter than my screaming.

Ask the group to think of another example following the set up above.

Slide 26

Anxiety Disorders

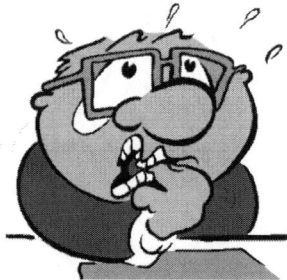

Slide 27

> ### Anxiety Disorders
>
> **Anxiety Disorders include a large number of conditions characterized by:**
>
> - Sense of apprehension
> - **Physiological symptoms – sweating, increased heart rate, increased rate of respiration**
> - Restlessness, fatigue, irritability, sleep disturbances, difficulty concentrating, muscle tension, personality changes.
> - **Lack of cause or situation does not warrant the extent of the reaction.**
>
> Hughes, 2005

There are several types of anxiety disorders. Symptoms vary depending on type. However, symptoms are generally:

Feelings of panic, fear, and uneasiness

Uncontrollable, obsessive thoughts

Repeated thoughts or flashbacks of traumatic experiences

Nightmares

Ritualistic behaviors, such as repeated hand washing

Problems sleeping

Cold or sweaty hands and/or feet

Shortness of breath

Palpitations

An inability to be still and calm

Dry mouth

Numbness or tingling in the hands or feet

Nausea

Muscle tension

Dizziness

Slide 28

> Anxiety Disorders
>
> ### Public Figures who have/had Anxiety Disorders
>
> - Barbara Streisand, Singer/Actor/Director
> - Nikola Tesla, Scientist/Inventor
> - Charles Darwin, Naturalist/Author
> - Johnny Depp, Actor
> - Neil Young, Musician

Slide 29

> **Types of Anxiety Disorders**
>
> **Among the anxiety disorders listed in the DSM 5 are;**
> - **Specific phobias:** Marked fear or anxiety about specific objects or situations, such as snakes, heights, flying, etc.
> - **Social anxiety disorder:** Marked fear or anxiety about one or more social situations in which the person is exposed to possible scrutiny by others.
> - **Panic Disorder:** Recurrent, unexpected panic attacks.
> - **Generalized anxiety disorder:** This disorder involves excessive, anxiety or worry occurring more days than not for at least 6 months, about a number of events or activities.
>
> DSM-5, 2013

Most people experience anxiety at different times such as when taking a test or going for a job interview. What differentiates the anxiety most people feel from anxiety disorders is the amount of impairment they cause to their every-day lives. The worry and fear people with anxiety disorders experience can seriously interfere in their lives on a daily basis.

MODULE IV

Slide 30

DSM 5 Symptoms of Generalized Anxiety Disorder	Presentation in Someone with IDD
A. Developmentally inappropriate and excessive fear or anxiety . Anxiety or worry associated with 3 or more of the following 6: · Restlessness · Easily fatigued · Difficulty concentrating · Irritability · Muscle tension · Sleep disturbances	• No adaptation from criteria in DSM 5

Anxiety Disorders

Diagnostic criteria that rely on subjective descriptions of symptoms are difficult to apply or detect in those with communication/cognitive problems. Therefore, incorporating behavioral equivalents within the context of cognitive, developmental and adaptive functioning, are proposed to facilitate accurate diagnosis. Excessive worry and difficulty controlling the worry may present in persons with oral communication skills as perseverative talk about the topic or issue creating the worry (self-talk or to others).

Slide 31

DSM 5 Symptoms of Generalized Anxiety Disorder	Presentation in Someone with IDD
B. Fear, anxiety or avoidance is persistent, lasting at least 4 wks	• Inapplicable in persons with Profound IDD (may mean it's diagnosis is not possible based on the person's limited ability for insight about thoughts or articulate thoughts and feelings).
C. Focus of Anxiety or worry	• No adaptation from DSM 5 for mild to moderate IDD. Difficulty to apply in persons with severe IDD. Inapplicable in persons with profound IDD.

Anxiety Disorders

Difficulty concentrating or mind going blank very difficult to apply in persons with Severe IDD and inapplicable for persons with Profound IDD. However, anxiety can be observed as self-injury (skin picking, pinching, etc.), pacing, inability to settle (restlessness), muscle rigidity (tension) and changes in sleep patterns, hyper-arousal, exaggerated startle responses, etc.

Slide 32

DSM 5 Symptoms of Generalized Anxiety Disorder	Presentation in Someone with IDD
E. Anxiety or worry causes clinically significant distress or impairment in social, academic, occupational, or other important areas of functioning.	• No adaptation from DSM 5
F. Anxiety or worry is not connected to the physiological effects of a substance, e.g., medication, drug or medical condition or not better explained by another disorder	• No adaptation from DSM 5

Anxiety Disorders

A person with IDD and anxiety may experience anxiety as a loss of skills that had been acquired, particularly for tasks with several steps in the sequence of completion like doing laundry, meal preparation, personal hygiene, etc.

Please note: The lists of symptoms are intended to be representative of the most common symptoms for Generalized Anxiety Disorders. These lists are not intended to be exhaustive or reflective of symptoms of other types of Mood Disorders.

Slide 33

Anxiety Disorders

Treatment Strategies

- **Psychotherapy with a focus on understanding and managing the disorder**
- Environmental and social modification
- **Social skill training**
- Regular exercise
- **Wellness based approaches**
- Learning stress management strategies
- **Anti-anxiety medication**

Hughes, 2005

A multi-faceted and multi-disciplinary treatment approach is recommended for generalized anxiety disorder. Generalized anxiety, when caught early, can be more easily treated successfully. The first line of treatment is likely to be medication treatment. This is to assist the individual to become more stable in order to benefit from other treatment and habilitative approaches. Once the person is stabilized then other supports can come into play, such as psycho-therapy and positive environmental adaptations and other positive supports as needed.

Slide 34

What symptoms of anxiety might look like for a person with IDD...

Set Up:	Set Off:	So I:	And I get or avoid:
Person has an Anxiety Disorder and an Autism Spectrum Disorder Low tolerance for frustration History of conflict with family Bullying type of personality	Family member interrupts routine	Begin to strip off my clothing	I am allowed to return to the routine I am comfortable following

Ask the group to think of another example following the set up above.

Slide 35

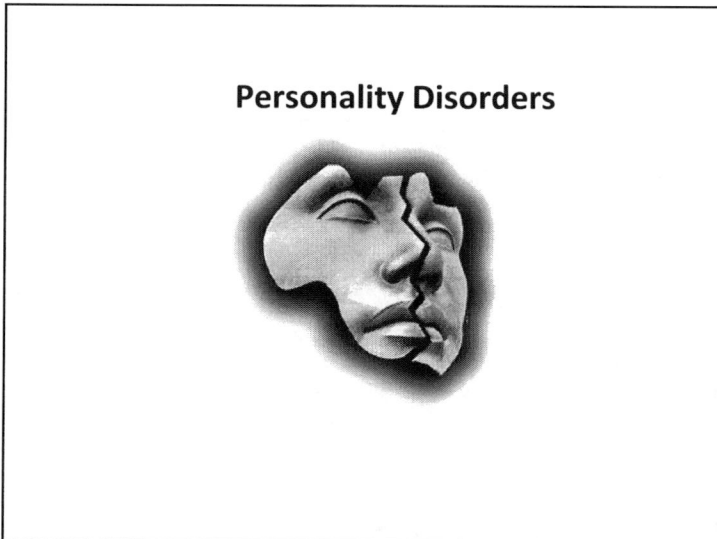

Personality Disorders

Slide 36

> **Personality Disorders**
>
> Personality Disorders are mental health disorders which cause difficulty perceiving and relating to situations and people including self. They are characterized by:
> - **Rigid and unhealthy patterns of thinking and behaving across situations.**
> - Frequent mood swings
> - **Stormy relationships**
> - Social isolation
> - **Angry outbursts**
> - Suspicion and mistrust of others
> - **Difficulty making friends**
> - A need for instant gratification
> - **Poor impulse control**
> - Alcohol or substance abuse

Important to note that many people with Borderline Personality Disorder (BPD) also have eating disorders, addiction issues, or depression and often have a history of trauma. Caution must be used to ensure that these issues are not masking the BPD and interfere with treatment decisions.

Slide 37

> **Personality Disorders**
>
> **Public Figures who have/had Personality Disorders**
>
> - Doug Ferrari – Comedian
> - Herschel Walker, NFL Player/Heisman Trophy Winner

Slide 38

Types of Personality Disorders

Among the different types of Personality Disorders listed in the DSM 5 are:

- **General Personality Disorder:** Enduring pattern of inner thoughts or behavior that deviates markedly from the expectations of the individual's culture
- **Paranoid Personality Disorder:** Pervasive distrust or suspiciousness of others such that their behavior is interpreted as malevolent
- **Dependent Personality Disorder:** Pervasive and excessive need to be taken care of that leads to submissive and clinging behavior and fear of separation

People with personality disorders experience patterns of behavior, mood, impulsiveness, and social interaction that can interfere with relationships with other people in their lives and create distress in those relationships. The symptoms of different personality disorders vary depending on type.

Slide 39

Personality Disorders

DSM 5 Symptoms of Borderline Personality Disorder (indicated by 5 or more of the following)	Presentation in Someone with IDD
1) Frantic efforts to avoid real or imagined abandonment.	• More reliant on caregivers than general population. Cultural sensitivities must also be considered.
2) Pattern of unstable and intense interpersonal relationships alternating between idealization and devaluation.	• No adaptation from DSM 5

M
O
D
U
L
E

I
V

Fear of abandonment can present as acts designed to "get rid of" others, unreasonable demands of staff at times, repeatedly calling family members on the phone, dramatic acts intended to keep the person from leaving. Patterns of unstable relationships can often be observed in the relationships between the person and their support staff, when applicable. The person may alternately choose one staff as a particular "favorite" on one occasion and adamantly refuse their involvement on other occasions.

Slide 40

	Personality Disorders
DSM 5 Symptoms of Borderline Personality Disorder	**Presentation in Someone with IDD**
3) Identity disturbance: markedly and persistently unstable self-image or sense of self.	• No adaptation – but note that expressions of self-image require fairly sophisticated verbal skills that may not be present in a person with IDD.
4) Impulsivity in at least 2 areas that are potentially self-damaging	• No adaptation from DSM-5 • Examples, spending, sexual activity, substance abuse, binge eating

People who have IDD can display identity disturbances by stating they are someone other than who they are.

Self-damage does not include suicidal or self-injury covered in criterion 5.

Slide 41

DSM 5 Symptoms of Borderline Personality Disorder	Presentation in Someone with IDD
5) Recurrent suicidal behavior, gestures, threats, or self-mutilating behavior	• No adaptation but note that self-injury can be a frequent problem for people with IDD and can be attributed to different causes.
6) Mood reactivity causing attentive instability.	• No adaptation from DSM 5 • e.g., irritability, intense episodic dysphoria/feeling of unease, anxiety usually lasting only a few hours

Personality Disorders

Mood reactivity presents as extreme changes in mood due to minor or non-existent issues.

Slide 42

DSM 5 Symptoms of Borderline Personality Disorder	Presentation in Someone with IDD
7) Chronic feelings of emptiness	• No adaptation - but note that expressions of feelings can require fairly sophisticated verbal skills that may not be present in a person with IDD
8) Inappropriate intense anger or difficulty controlling anger	• No adaptation – but note that anger problems are frequently noted for people with IDD.
9) Temporary paranoia brought on by stress or severe symptoms of dissociation	• No adaptation from DSM 5

Personality Disorders

Poor anger control can include both verbal and physical acts of aggression including self-harm.

MODULE IV

Please note: The lists of symptoms are intended to be representative of the most common symptoms for Borderline Personality Disorder. These lists are not intended to be exhaustive or reflective of symptoms of other types of Personality Disorders.

Slide 43

Personality Disorders

Treatment Strategies
- Individual or group therapy – cognitive and dialectic behavior therapy are most effective
- Environmental and social modification
- Social skill training
- Regular exercise
- Positive Behavioral Supports
- Psychotropic medication can be helpful for primary presenting symptoms.
- Emotional regulation
- Learning stress management strategies/stress tolerance
- Positive identity development

Hughes, 2006

Therapies should focus on: helping the person understand their illness; developing skills to control impulsivity; identifying ways to recognize and change negative thinking.

Slide 44

Set Up:	Set Off:	So I:	And I get or avoid:
Borderline Personality Disorder Lots of staff turnover Placed with people who are lower functioning Wants to "be" staff New manager creates conflict on the team	Staff are arguing back and forth	Make the divide between staff bigger escalating their argument.	I get to watch the conflict and drama that result.

What symptoms of Borderline Personality Disorder might look like for a person with IDD...

Ask the group to think of another example following the set up above.
For example:

Set Up:	Depression Low coping skills Not that interested in work Just got dumped by "boyfriend"
Set Off:	Cued regarding going to work
So I:	Ignore cue and become aggressive
And I get or avoid:	Avoid going to work. Work and paycheck used to be an incentive, but due to depression formerly preferred events are not preferred.

Slide 45

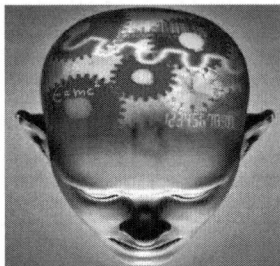

Schizophrenia and other Psychosis

Slide 46

Psychosis

- **The defining characteristics of psychosis are delusions, hallucinations, and disorganized speech or behavior.**

- There is evidence that current diagnostic criteria from DSM 5 can be used reliably for people with IDD but behavioral disturbances do seem more significant for people with Severe to Profound IDD than with Mild IDD.

When diagnosing psychosis, ruling out any medical conditions that can cause psychosis should be among the first steps.

In people with IDD, caution must be paid to ensure that self-talk, imaginary friends, fantasy play and beliefs, and beliefs based on faulty learning, all of which are common behaviors for people with IDD, are not misidentified as hallucinations or delusions. (Hughes, 2006)

Slide 47

> **Psychosis**
>
> ### Public Figures who have/had Psychosis
>
> - John Forbes Nash, Mathematician
> - Lionel Aldridge, NFL Player (Super Bowl champion)
> - Peter Green, Blues Musician/Founder Fleetwood Mac
> - Jack Kerouac, Author
> - Zelda Sayre Fitzgerald, American Novelist

Slide 48

> **Types of Psychosis**
>
> **Among the Psychotic Disorders listed in the DSM 5 are;**
>
> - Schizoaffective Disorder
> - Delusional Disorder
> - Schizophreniform Disorder
> - Substance/Medication Induced Psychotic Disorder

Psychotic disorders are characterized by abnormal thinking, perceptions and loss of touch with reality. Main symptoms are hallucinations and delusions. Hallucinations are false perceptions e.g., seeing something that isn't there, hearing a voice that isn't there. Delusions are false beliefs, such as believing one has superhuman strength when one does not.

Slide 49

Psychosis

DSM 5 Symptoms Of Schizophrenia	Presentation in Someone with IDD
A) Two or more of the following present for a significant portion of a 1 month period: · Delusions · Hallucinations · Disorganized speech · Grossly disorganized behavior · Negative symptoms, i.e., affect flattening, newly evidenced inability to speak, general lack of motivation or desire to pursue meaningful goals.	• No adaptation – note that developmentally appropriate self-talk, imaginary friends, fantasy play, and beliefs based on faulty learning can be confused with hallucinations and delusions.

Some research suggests that current estimates put the risk of schizophrenia in individuals with intellectual/developmental disability at around 3%, compared with a lifetime population risk of around 1%. (Hemmings, 2006)

Over their lifetime of contact with psychiatric services, individuals with a dual diagnosis ultimately diagnosed with schizophrenia were more likely initially to have been given diagnoses of paranoid psychoses; personality disorders; psychotic and non-psychotic organic disorders; acute reaction to stress or adjustment reaction; specific delays in development; disturbance of conduct; neurotic disorders; and depressive disorders. Evidently, based on the prevalence of misdiagnosis of psychotic disorders, schizophrenia in particular, symptoms of psychotic disorders in people with intellectual/developmental disability may present in atypical ways making it difficult to make an accurate diagnosis.

Slide 50

DSM 5 Symptoms of Schizophrenia	Presentation in Someone with IDD
B. Level of functioning in one or more major areas, such as work, interpersonal relations, or self-care is markedly below the level achieved prior to onset	• No Adaptation – but note that functional areas are dependent upon functioning level for the person.
C. Duration – continuous signs of the disturbance exist for at least six months.	• No adaptation from DSM 5 level of skill markedly below level achieved prior to onset for example, self-care skills, interpersonal relations,

Psychosis

A key point to remember when diagnosing psychosis is the cognitive level of functioning of the person with IDD. Impairment in level of functioning related to psychosis must take into consideration the level of functioning related to the level of IDD.

Slide 51

DSM IV-TR Symptoms of Schizophrenia	Presentation in Someone with ID
D) Schizoaffective disorder and depressive bipolar disorder with psychotic features have been ruled out	• No adaptation from DSM-5
E) The disturbance is not due to direct physiological effects of substance or general medical condition	• No adaptation from DSM-5

Psychosis

MODULE IV

Schizoaffective disorder is largely a disorder of mood and thought. Common symptoms are auditory hallucinations, paranoid thinking, and disorganized speech and thinking.

Symptoms of depressive bipolar disorder include irritability, guilt, unpredictable mood swings, restlessness, slowed speech and movement, and increased sleep. It also involves an increased tendency to lose contact with reality (psychosis).

Slide 52

	Psychosis
DSM 5 Symptoms Of Schizophrenia	**Presentation in Someone with IDD**
F. If there is a history of Autism Spectrum Disorder or a Communication Disorder of childhood onset, the additional diagnosis of schizophrenia is made only if prominent delusions or hallucinations, in addition to other required symptoms of schizophrenia, are also present for at least one month	• No adaptation from DSM 5

DSM-5 2013

Clinicians should be aware that any significant change in behavior can signify the possibility of psychosis, e.g., increase in self-injury, aggressive behavior or atypical behavior for the person.

Please note: The lists of symptoms are intended to be representative of the most common symptoms for Schizophrenia. They are not intended to be exhaustive or reflective of symptoms of other types of Psychoses.

Slide 53

> Psychosis
>
> ### Treatment Strategies
>
> - Adhering to a daily routine
> - **Social skill training**
> - Vocational Training
> - **Positive Support Strategies**
> - Education regarding schizophrenia
> - **Recreation Therapy**
> - Antipsychotic medication

There is evidence to indicate that psycho-social or cognitive therapy, and peer support groups can be effective in conjunction with medications.

Slide 54

> **What symptoms of Psychosis might look like for a person with IDD...**
>
> | Set Up: | Set Off: | So I: | And I get or avoid: |
> |---|---|---|---|
> | Psychosis

Lives with 3 other people with IDD | Auditory hallucination at breakfast | Yell back to "the voice" | Roommates take their coffee out to the porch |

Ask the group to think of another example following the set up above.

References: Module IV

American Psychiatric Association. (2013). *Diagnostic and statistical manual of mental disorders* (5th ed.). Washington, DC: Author.

Beers, M.H., & Berkow, R. (1999). *The Merck manual of diagnosis and therapy.* Wiley.

Deb, S., Thomas, M. & Bright, C. (2001). Mental disorder in adults with intellectual disability: prevalence of functional psychiatric illness among a community-based population aged between 16 and 64 years. *Journal of Intellectual Disability Research, 45,* 495–505.

Fletcher, R., Loschen, E., Stavrakaki, C., & First, M. (Eds.). (2007). *Diagnostic manual – Intellectual disability (DM-ID): A Clinical guide for diagnosis of mental disorders in persons with intellectual disability.* Kingston, NY: NADD Press.

Hemmings, C.P. (2006). Schizophrenia spectrum disorders in people with intellectual disabilities. *Current Opinion in Psychiatry, 19,* 470 -4.

Hughes, E.E. (2006). *The dual diagnosis primer: A training manual for family members, case managers, advocates, guardians and direct support professionals.* Kingston, NY: NADD Press.

Laman, D. S., & Reiss, S. (1987). Social skill deficiencies associated with depressed mood of mentally retarded adults. *American Journal of Mental Deficiency, 92,* 224-229.

Matson, J. L., Barrett, R., & Helsel, W. J. (1988). Depression in mentally retarded children. *Research in Developmental Disabilities, 9,* 39-46.

Morgan, V.A., Leonard, H., Bourke, J., Assen, J. (2006). Intellectual disability co-occurring with schizophrenia and other psychiatric illness: population-based study. *The British Journal of Psychiatry, 193,* 364-372.

From the DM-ID to the DM-ID-2

Slide 1

> # Module V
>
> **From the DM-ID**
> **To the**
> **DM-ID-2**

Slide 2

> **This module contains information about the DM-ID and the DM-ID-2 and how they assist in the diagnostic process for persons with IDD.**

Slide 3

Learning Objectives

- Describe the purpose of the DM-ID-2
- Identify 3 types of modifications of the DSM criteria which are contained in the DM-ID-2
- Describe the significance of the cognitive developmental level in relationship to criteria subsets
- Articulate why the DSM system does not apply to people who have language deficits

---

Slide 4

Limitations of DSM System

- Diagnostic Overshadowing (Reiss, et al, 1982)

- Applicability of established diagnostic systems is increasingly suspect as the severity of IDD increases (Rush & Frances, 2000)

- DSM System relies on self report of signs and symptoms (DSM-IV-TR, DSM-5)

Until the development of the DM-ID, clinicians relied on the DSM system to diagnose psychiatric disorders in persons with IDD. However, there are significant limitations in using the DSM system for persons who have IDD.

The concept of "diagnostic overshadowing" makes it difficult for clinicians to identify a mental illness in persons with IDD. Diagnostic overshadowing refers to the process of over-attributing a patient's symptoms to a particular condition, resulting in key comorbid conditions being undiagnosed and untreated. Diagnostic overshadowing was originally described in people with developmental disabilities, where their psychiatric symptoms and behaviors were falsely attributed to their disability, leaving any comorbid psychiatric illness undiagnosed. Increasingly, research has also shown that comorbid medical conditions are often "diagnostically overshadowed" by the presence of a prior psychiatric disorder or developmental disability diagnosis.

The DSM system relies on self-report of the client. The person expresses to the clinician his or her feelings, thoughts, and emotions. Many people with IDD, especially those with limited verbal skills, are challenged in their ability to give a self-report of signs and symptoms.

The DSM system can apply effectively for people who have good expressive and receptive language skills However, the DSM system has limited application for people who have language deficits.

Slide 5

```
                                                        DM–ID
                        Diagnostic Manual – Intellectual Disabilities

                                    Developed By

              National Association for the Dually Diagnosed

                                        (NADD)

                                  In association with

                        American Psychiatric Association

                                        (APA)

              Partial Funding from the Joseph P. Kennedy, Jr. Foundation
                        Published by the NADD Press, 2007
```

The DM-ID was developed by NADD in association with the APA and published in 2007. The work on the DM-ID began in 1997, and it took ten years to develop this diagnostic manual.

There were approximately 100 psychiatrists and other clinicians from around the world who worked on the development of the DM-ID using an expert consensus model.

Developing the DM-ID was a major project and was partially funded by the Joseph P. Kennedy Jr. Foundation.

Slide 6

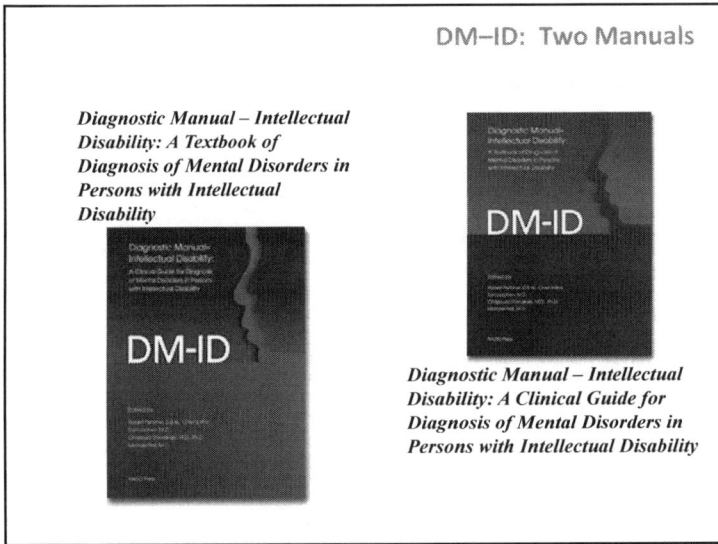

Actually two diagnostic manuals were developed. The *Diagnostic Manual – Intellectual Disability: A Textbook of Diagnosis of Mental Disorders in Persons with Intellectual Disability* was developed first. This is a rather large book with over 550 pages.

After that was done, a large number of peer reviewers and the NADD International Advisory Committee suggested the development of a clinical manual that would be easily accessible to both psychiatrists as well as primary care physicians. A second diagnostic manual entitled *Diagnostic Manuel – Intellectual Disability: A Clinical Guide for Diagnosis of Mental Disorders in Persons with Intellectual Disability* was developed based on these recommendations. Everything that is in the 350 plus pages clinical guide is also in the textbook.

The textbook has a great deal of background information, a review of the research for each diagnostic category, as well as a section on pathogenesis and etiology for each diagnostic category.

All of the diagnoses, diagnostic subcategories, and criteria modifications are identical in both books. Both books can be used to diagnose a specific psychiatric disorder in persons with IDD.

Slide 7

Description of DM-ID

- An adaptation to the *DSM-IV-TR*

- Designed to facilitate a more accurate psychiatric diagnosis

- Based on Expert Consensus Model

- Covers all major diagnostic categories as defined in *DSM-IV-TR*

The DM-ID is a modification or an adaptation to the DSM-IV-TR. It uses the same diagnostic categories as are found in the DSM-IV-TR. However, there are adaptations to criteria subsets, as warranted. With the release of the DSM 5, NADD will now spearhead an update of the DM-ID to correspond with the new guidelines.

The DM-ID was designed to facilitate a more accurate psychiatric diagnosis in persons with IDD.

It was based on an expert consensus model. Each diagnostic category was developed by a group of experts, represented by between two to eight clinicians and academicians from around the globe. Thus, approximately 100 people were involved in the development of the DM-ID.

All of the diagnostic categories that are defined in the DSM-IV-TR are also in the DM-ID. Additionally, the codification system, used for insurance purposes, are the same in the DSM-IV-TR as they are in the DM-ID.

Slide 8

Description of DM-ID (continued)

- **Provides information to help with diagnostic process**

- Addresses pathoplastic effect of IDD on psychopathology (how the disorder is manifested in people with IDD)

- **Designed with a developmental perspective to help clinicians to recognize symptom profiles in adults and children with IDD**

The DM-ID has a wealth of information in each diagnostic category to assist the clinician at arriving at an accurate diagnosis.

Each diagnostic category describes how the psychiatric disorder can be manifested in persons with IDD.

A developmental perspective is emphasized throughout the DM-ID to assist the clinician to recognize psychiatric disorders in persons with IDD. The expression of a specific psychiatric disorder can differ depending on the level of functioning and IQ level. The DM-ID informs the reader of these differences for each psychiatric disorder.

Slide 9

Description of DM-ID (continued)

- **Empirically-based approach to identify specific psychiatric disorders in persons with IDD**

- **Provides state-of-the-art information about mental disorders in persons with IDD**

- **Provides adaptations of criteria, where appropriate**

The Textbook offers a comprehensive review of the research literature for each diagnostic category.

Both manuals have a wealth of information about how to apply a DSM diagnosis for persons with IDD.

In the DM-ID, there are adaptations or modifications to criteria subsets from the DSM-IV-TR.

Slide 10

**Field Study of the
Clinical Usefulness of the DM-ID**

<u>Table 1</u>: Clinician Impressions by Level of Intellectual Disability (%YES)

Item	Level of Intellectual Disability		
	Mild N=305	Moderate N=237	Severe/ Profound N=285
Was the DM-ID easy to use (user friendly)?	72.4	68.6	62.6
Did you find the DM-ID clinically useful in the diagnosis of this patient?	74.9	67.8	66.0
Did DM-ID allow you to arrive at an appropriate psychiatric diagnosis for this patient?	85.6	83.3	80.2
Did DM-ID allow you to come up with a more specific diagnosis than you would have with the *DSM-IV-TR*?	36.1	38.0	35.9
Did DM-ID help you avoid using the NOS category?	63.2	63.3	54.9

Fletcher, et a., 2009

Field study research was conducted to identify the clinical usefulness of the DM-ID. The research was conducted on 827 different individuals. There were 90 clinicians involved in this research study. The study was conducted in 11 different countries. Overall, clinicians involved in testing the DM-ID found it clinically useful.

This chart illustrates that there was a fairly even distribution of clients involved from the mild level, moderate level, and severe/profound level.

The chart also illustrates that the majority of clinicians found the DM-ID to be:
- user-friendly
- clinically useful
- helpful to arrive at an appropriate diagnosis
- helpful to avoid using the NOS category

The research data indicates that the DM-ID is a useful tool in helping to arrive at a more accurate psychiatric diagnosis.

Slide 11

> ### The Publication of the DSM-5
> ### Necessitates
> ### Revision of the DM-ID
>
> # THE DM-ID-2

The APA released a revision of the *Diagnostic and Statistical Manual* in May, 2013 (*DSM-5*). With the release of the *DSM-5* it becomes important that the *DM-ID* be revised to correspond the *DSM-5* and to incorporate the changes in the *DSM-5*. There are many changes and revisions in this edition. It will be important to incorporate these changes into a future volume of the *DM-ID* to insure the most accurate psychiatric diagnoses for individuals with IDD.

NADD has embarked on a multi-year project to revise the *DM-ID* to correspond to the *DSM-5*. Dr. Robert Fletcher is Chief Editor, and Dr. Sally-Ann Cooper and Dr. Jarrett Barnhill are Co-Editors. NADD will again use an expert-consensus model, with work groups of 4-8 experts for each of 26 diagnostic categories. The *DM-ID-2* will use the same diagnostic categories identified in the *DSM-5*.

Slide 12

DM-ID-2
Two Special Added-Value Chapters

- **Assessment and Diagnostic Procedures**

- **Behavioral Phenotype of Genetic Disorders**

The DM-ID-2 offers two chapters that are not part of the DSM-5. One is on assessment and diagnostic procedures and the other is on behavioral phenotypes of genetic disorders.

The chapter on assessment and diagnostic procedures discusses the types of historical information needed for an effective mental health evaluation.

The chapter on behavioral phenotypes and genetic disorders discusses twelve commonly found genetic disorders and the corresponding behavioral phenotypes associated with each disorder.

Slide 13

> Assessment and Diagnostic
> Procedures Chapter
>
> **Psychiatric diagnosis is a challenge**
>
> **Need to rely on multiple sources for information**
>
> **Need to understand their challenges**
>
> **Be empathetic**
>
> Hurley et al. in prep.

This valuable chapter includes information on how to conduct a mental health assessment in persons with IDD.

Psychiatric diagnosis and treatment is always challenging due to the complexity of human nature, cultural differences, male-female differences, personality and neuropsychological abilities as well as other ecological social and historical factors. There are no "lab" tests to help us diagnose a patient. When the patient is a person with a specific neurodevelopmental disorder, such as intellectual disability, the process of diagnosis and treatment is that much more complicated.

The practitioner cannot accept the discourse as reliable and, therefore, must use multiple sources of information to assist in the evaluation process. Under the best of circumstances, the diagnosis can be quite provisional. The aim of the clinician who cares for a person with intellectual disability must be to try to see the world through their eyes; understand the difficulties imposed by developmental delay; be sympathetic to their difficulties navigating modern life; and understand their relationships and supports. Unlike a typical person, those with intellectual disability are at great disadvantage in speaking for themselves in all area of life, and none so obvious as the psychiatric diagnostic interview.

Slide 14

Special Considerations

- Use language that can be understood

- Confirm understanding

Establishing Chief Complaint and History

- Ask client

- Ask other individuals

- Obtain historical information

The mental health clinician must exercise special care in several areas when interacting with an individual who has intellectual disability. First, the clinician must use language that is understandable to the individual and needs to verify the individual's comprehension. Because clinicians customarily talk rapidly, and use complex language in long sentences, individuals with intellectual disability can be at a disadvantage during the interview. The clinician should make the following adjustments: (a) Use very simple vocabulary words, (b) create short sentences, (c) ask one simple question at a time, (d) wait for the answer before proceeding, (e) check back with the individual for confirmation that he or she has correctly understood the question and (f) use visuals to assist understanding and engagement. For individual with little or no language, using nonverbal strategies or body language will facilitate the therapeutic engagement and enrich the psychiatric evaluation.

The clinician should ask family and direct support professionals about the onset and chronology of changes in any or all of the following: school, day services, residential services, and family life. This information, acquired not only from the individual but--more importantly—from all other possible sources, will comprise the history of present illness. It is important not only to elicit the presenting problem, but to determine who has defined the problem, how long it has been observed, in what environments it is observed, and—if longstanding in nature—why evaluation is being sought at this time. It is crucial that the person or persons making the referral for evaluation are present to explain their concerns (Levitas, Hurley, & Pary, 2001). It is equally crucial to have available sources from which, or by which, the individual's premorbid functioning can be described.

Slide 15

DM-ID-2
Assessment and Diagnostic
Procedures Chapter

Historical Information

Hurley, et al. in pres

It is important for the clinician to obtain historical information as part of the mental health assessment. In addition to a thorough history and mental status examination, a review of prior records is an important part of conducting an assessment from a bio-psycho-social perspective. For example, the assessment should include historical information about early childhood, school, family relationships, substance abuse, trauma, medical, mental health, IQ testing, occupational, as well as present situation.

MODULE V

Slide 16

Behavioral Phenotype of
Genetic Disorders Chapter

Angelman Syndrome

Chromosome 15q112-131
Duplication Syndrome

Down Syndrome

Fetal Alcohol Syndrome

Fragile-X Syndrome

Phenylketonuria

Prader-Willi Syndrome

Rubenstein-Taybi Syndrome

Smith-Magenis Syndrome

Tuberous Sclerosis Complex

Velocardiofacial Syndrome

Williams Syndrome

The phenotype of a genetic syndrome is the set of physical characteristics produced by a genetic abnormality or genotype as discussed in Module I. The most widely known example is the easily recognized face of a person with Down Syndrome.

The phrase "behavioral phenotype" denotes a set of behaviors that are genetically determined and associated with a particular genetic disorder. A behavioral phenotype is the specific and characteristic behavioral repertoire exhibited by persons with a specific genetic disorder.

This chapter lists twelve genetic disorders and their associated behavioral phenotypes. For each of the twelve disorders there is information on physical findings, diagnosis, cognition, behavioral, and associated mental health disorders.

Slide 17

| DM-ID-2 |
| Behavioral Phenotype of Genetic Disorders Chapter |
| Phenotype and Behavioral Phenotype for |
| Down Syndrome |

Phenotype	Small head, mouth; upward slant to eyes; epicanthal folds; broad neck; hypothyroidism; hearing loss; visual impairments; cardiac problems; gastro-intestinal; orthopedic, and skin disorders; obesity	
Behavioral Phenotype	Childhood	Oppositional and defiant; attention-deficit/hyperactivity disorder (ADHD): social, charming personality "stereotype"; self-talk
	Adulthood	Depressive disorders; obsessive-compulsive disorder; other anxiety disorders; dementia of the Alzheimer's type; mental disorders associated with hypothyroidism; atypical psychoses; self-talk

Levitas, et al. in press

This table is an example of a phenotype and behavioral phenotype for Down syndrome. The cluster of characteristic behaviors in a person with Down syndrome is differentiated between childhood behaviors and adult behaviors.

A key value in understanding behavioral phenotypes is that it aids in the diagnostic process. The behavioral phenotypes provide information that, when combined with other sources of information, aids in the diagnostic process.

Combining behavioral phenotypes with other sources of information provides the clinicians with important pieces of the complex diagnostic puzzle.

MODULE V

Slide 18

DM-ID-2
Diagnostic Chapter Structure

- **Review of Diagnostic Criteria**
  - **General description of the disorder**
  - **Summary of *DSM-5* criteria**

- Issues related to diagnosis in people with IDD

- **Review of Literature/Research**
  - **Evaluating level of evidence**

There is a lot of consistency and uniformity throughout the DM-ID-2. There are categories and sub-categories that are listed in each of the diagnostic chapters. For example, each chapter has a section on:
  - Review of Diagnostic Criteria
  - Issues related to diagnosis in people with IDD
  - Review of Literature/Research (Textbook only)

Slide 19

Application of Diagnostic Criteria to People with IDD

- General considerations

- **Adults with Mild to Moderate IDD**

- Adults with Severe or Profound IDD

- **Children and adolescents with IDD**

All of the diagnostic chapters follow a consistent outline of information. The DM-ID-2 has a section for each diagnostic category on the application of diagnostic criteria to people with IDD. In addition to general considerations, this section differentiates adults with mild to moderate levels of IDD and addresses the manifestation of a specific disorder for adults who have severe or profound IDD. The manifestation of a particular psychiatric disorder can be manifested differently in children and adolescents with IDD. Therefore, there is also a subsection for each diagnostic category that articulates the expression of that disorder in children and adolescents with IDD.

MODULE V

Slide 20

The DM-ID-2 Textbook has a section for each diagnostic category concerning etiology and pathogenesis. Under this section there are subcategories of risk factors including biological, psychosocial, and genetic syndromes. This information provides the clinician with a better understanding of the nature and source of the psychiatric disorder. Assembling this information aids in the diagnostic process.

Slide 21

DM-ID-2
(continued)

Diagnostic Criteria

DSM-IV-TR Criteria	Applying Criteria to Mild-Moderate IDD	Applying Criteria to Severe-Profound IDD

At the end of most diagnostic chapters there is a chart with three columns:

- the left column has the DSM-IV-TR criteria and criteria subsets

- the middle column offers information about applying the criteria for persons with mild/moderate levels of IDD

- the right column offers information about applying the criteria for persons with severe/profound levels of IDD

Slide 22

DM-ID-2
(continued)

Diagnostic Criteria

DSM-IV-TR Criteria	Applying Criteria for IDD (Mild to Profound)

There are a few charts that list the DSM-5 criteria on the left side and the right side is a column for applying criteria for persons with mild to profound levels of IDD.

Slide 23

```
                                              DM-ID-2
                                              (continued)

              Modifications of the DSM-5 Criteria

          1.  Addition of symptom equivalents

          2.  Omission of symptoms

          3.  Changes in symptom count

          4.  Modification of symptom duration
```

The DM-ID-2 has seven different modifications of the DSM-5 criteria.

1. Addition of symptom equivalents – these are observed behaviors that are equivalent to self reports as identified in the DSM system.

2. Omission of symptoms – these are symptoms that do not exist or cannot be identified in persons with IDD

3. Changes in symptom count – this indicates the frequency of a symptom that is required to meet a diagnostic category

4. Modification of symptom duration – This indicates the length of time a symptom has to be present in order to meet the diagnostic criteria.

MODULE V

Slide 24

DM-ID-2
(continued)

Modifications of the DSM-5 Criteria

5. Modification of age requirements

6. Addition of explanatory notes

7. Criteria Sets that do not apply

(The DM-ID-2 has seven different modifications of the DSM-5 criteria – continued)

5. Modification of age requirements – this indicates a change in the age of a person with regard to a particular criteria of a diagnostic category. This is to take into consideration the developmental perspective of the individual with IDD.

6. Addition of explanatory notes – there are many explanatory notes in the context of criteria subsets that are intended to communicate a criteria adaptation. An explanatory note is provided in situations where there was insufficient research data, but sufficient clinical expert consensus to explain a change in criteria without an official modification of the criteria subset.

7. Criteria Sets that do not apply – in the DM-ID-2 there are occasionally criteria in the DSM system that do not apply to people with IDD. These criteria sets that do not apply are identified in the section under schizophrenia and delusional disorder in persons with severe/profound levels of IDD.

Slide 25

<table>
<tr><td colspan="2" align="center">Modification of DSM-5 Criteria
Change in Count and Symptom Equivalent
Major Depressive Disorder</td></tr>
<tr><td align="center">DSM-5 Criteria</td><td align="center">Applying Criteria for Mild
to Profound IDD</td></tr>
<tr>
<td>A. Five or more of the following symptoms have been present during the same 2 week period and represent a change from previous functioning. At least one of the symptoms is either (1) depressed mood or (2) loss of interest or pleasure.</td>
<td>A. Four or more symptoms have been present during the same 2 week period and represent a change from previous functioning. At least one of the symptoms is either (1) depressed mood or (2) loss of interest or pleasure or (3) irritable mood</td>
</tr>
</table>

Major depressive disorder – in this diagnostic category there are changes in the symptom count as well as changes in symptom equivalence. Specifically, the DM-ID-2 has four or more symptoms … compared to five or more in the DSM-5. This is an example of change in symptom count.

There is also an addition to symptom equivalent as irritable mood was added.

These changes may appear subtle on the surface, but have significant importance with regard to the diagnostic process of identifying major depressive disorder in persons with IDD.

MODULE V

243

Slide 26

DSM-5 Criteria	Applying Criteria for Individuals with IDD
A. There is a pervasive pattern of disregard for and violation of the rights of others occurring since age 15 years, as indicated by three (or more) of the following:	A. There is a pervasive pattern of disregard for and violation of the rights of others occurring since age 18 years, as indicated by three (or more) of the following:
B. The individual is at least age 18 years	B. The individual is at least age 21 years
C. There is evidence of Conduct Disorder with the onset before age 15 years	C. There is evidence of Conduct Disorder with onset before age 18 years

Modifications of DSM-5 Criteria
Modification of Age

Antisocial Personality Disorder

DSM-5 ... (source)

Antisocial Personality Disorder

There are changes in modification of age in the three criteria subsets. These changes reflect the cognitive developmental level of the individual with IDD.

Slide 27

<table>
<tr><td colspan="2" align="right">Modification of Criteria
Addition of Explanatory Note</td></tr>
<tr><td colspan="2" align="center">Manic Episode</td></tr>
<tr>
<td>DSM-IV-TR Criteria</td>
<td>Applying Criteria for
Mild to Profound IDD</td>
</tr>
<tr>
<td>A. A distinct period of abnormally persistently elevated, expansive or irritable mood, lasting at least 1 week (or any duration if hospitalization is necessary)</td>
<td>A. No adaptation.
Note: Observers may report that the individual with IDD: has loud inappropriate laughing or singing, is excessively giddy or silly; is intrusive, getting into other's space; and smiles excessively and in ways that are not appropriate to the social context. Elated mood may be alternating with irritable mood</td>
</tr>
</table>

DM-ID 2007

Manic Episode

This is an example of the addition of an explanatory note. The explanatory note is nearly the same as an adaptation to the DSM-5 criteria. The only difference is that the explanatory note is based on clinical experience rather than research data. The explanatory note communicates to the reader specific behaviors that are characteristic in persons with IDD who experience a manic episode.

MODULE V

Slide 28

The Future

DM-ID 2

In Development

Edited By:

Robert Fletcher , DSW, ACSW, NADD-CC

Jarrett Barnhill, M.D., DFAPA, FAACAP

Sally Ann Cooper, BSc (Hons), MB, BS, MD, FRCPsych

References: Module V

Fletcher, R., Havercamp, S., Ruedrich, S., Benson, B., Barnhill, J., Cooper, S-A., & Stavrakaki, C. (2009). Clinical usefulness of the diagnostic manual-intellectual disability to mental disorders in persons with intellectual disability: Results from a brief field survey. *The Journal of Clinical Psychiatry, 70(7)*, 967-974.

Fletcher, R., Barnhill, J., & Cooper, S-A. (in press). *Diagnostic Manual – Intellectual Disability (DM-ID-2): A Textbook of Diagnosis of Mental Disorders in Persons with Intellectual Disability* (2nd ed.). Kingston, N.Y.: NADD Press.

Fletcher, R, Loschen, E, Stavrakaki, C, & First, M. (2007). *Diagnostic manual – Intellectual disability: A textbook of diagnosis of mental disorders in persons with intellectual disability*. Kingston, NY: NADD Press.

Hurley, A.D., Levitas, A., Luiselli, J.K, Moss, S., Bradley, E, & Bailey, N. (in press). Assessment and diagnostic procedures. In R. Fletcher, J. Barnhill, & S-A. Cooper (Eds.), *Diagnostic Manual – Intellectual Disability (DM-ID-2): A Textbook of Diagnosis of Mental Disorders in Persons with Intellectual Disability* (2nd ed.). Kingston, N.Y.: NADD Press.

Levitas, A., Dykens, E., Finucane, B., E., Simon, Schuster, M., Kates, W., Oslewski, Dykens, E., & Danker, N. (in press). Behavioral phenotypes of neurodevelopmental disorders. In R. Fletcher, J. Barnhill, & S-A. Cooper (Eds.), *Diagnostic Manual – Intellectual Disability (DM-ID-2): A Textbook of Diagnosis of Mental Disorders in Persons with Intellectual Disability* (2nd ed.). Kingston, N.Y.: NADD Press.

Reiss, S., Levitan, G.W., Szyszko, J. (1982). Emotional disturbance and mental retardation: diagnostic overshadowing. *American Journal of Mental Deficiencies, 86(6)*, 567-74.

Rush, A.J., Frances, A. (Eds.). (2000). Treatment of psychiatric and behavioural problems in mental retardation (Special Issue). *American Journal of Mental Retardation, 105(3)*, 1-71.

MODULE V

M O D U L E   V

Support Strategies

Slide 1

Module VI

Support Strategies

Slide 2

Support Strategies

In this module, we will discuss the following advanced support strategies:

1. Positive Behavior Supports

2. Communication Tone

3. Environmental

4. Choice and self determination

5. Relaxation techniques

6. Verbal strategies

Slide 3

> # Learning Objectives
>
> - Discuss 5 principles for achieving a therapeutic relationship
> - Name 3 special considerations when conducting therapy with people who have IDD/MI
> - Describe 5 predictable crises
> - Summarize 3 crisis management strategies
> - Describe the main characteristics and components of Positive Behavior Supports
> - Describe the importance of communication and setting tone when supporting a person with IDD
> - List and describe verbal and non-verbal de-escalation support strategies

Slide 4

> Positive Behavior Supports
>
> ## Positive Behavior Support
>
> (PBS) involves the changing situations and events that people with problem behaviors experience in order to reduce the likelihood of their occurrence and increase social, personal, and professional quality in their lives.
>
> Carr & Sidener, 2002

Positive behavior support is an approach to behavior intervention largely derived from applied behavior analysis (ABA) that uses a system to understand what maintains an individual's challenging behaviors and a holistic, person-centered approach to addressing them. People's inappropriate behaviors are difficult to change because they are functional; they serve a purpose for the person. These behaviors are supported by reinforcement in the environment.

Positive behavior support (PBS) developed in the 1980s and 1990s as an approach to enhance quality of life and minimize challenging behavior (Carr & Sidener, 2002).

Slide 5

Positive Behavior Support

What does PBS Consider?

- Values about the rights and dignity of people who have disabilities and self-determination
- Practical science about how learning and behavior change occur
- Biomedical concerns
- Lifestyle concerns
- Changes in systems of support
- Team-based approaches

Carr & Sidener, 2002

Carr & Sidner (2002) described PBS as "an applied science that uses educational methods to expand an individual's behavior repertoire and systems change methods to redesign an individual's living environment to first enhance the individual's quality of life and, second, to minimize his or her problem behavior." It was developed out of an identified need to eliminate aversive consequences with people who have intellectual/developmental disabilities.

Human rights are in the forefront of considering how to address problem behaviors. Many problem behaviors are learned, and as such teaching new skills is often the most important intervention. Other problem behaviors are caused by physical problems such as dental pain. Idle hands are the devil's work tools, and bored people might seek entertainment with actions we consider problems.

Slide 6

> **Positive Behavior Supports**
>
> ### Considerations (continued)
>
> - Decrease negative behaviors
> - Support appropriate behavior
> - Focus on improving environment, not "fixing" people
> - Quality of life enhancement
> - Increase learning and independence
> - Successful input and collaboration from those closest to the person and the person themselves
> - Cooperation across disciplines

PBS values include commitments to respect for the individual, meaningful outcomes, dignity, normalization, inclusion in the community, person-centered planning, self-determination, and stakeholder participation, among others.

Slide 7

> **Positive Behavior Supports**
>
> ### Components of a PBS Approach
>
> - Functional Assessment
>
> - Comprehensive Intervention
>
> - Focus on Quality of Life and Wellness

Components of a functional assessment include:
- A clear description of the problem behaviors
- Events, times, and situations that predict when behaviors will and will not occur (i.e., setting events)
- Consequences that maintain the problem behaviors (the function)
- Summary statements or hypotheses
- Direct observation data to support the hypotheses

Interventions include: 1) proactive strategies for changing the environment so triggering events are removed, 2) teaching new skills that replace problem behaviors, 3) eliminating or minimizing natural reinforcement for problem behavior, and 4) maximizing clear reinforcement for appropriate behavior.

The underlying focus is overall enhancement of the quality of life of the person with a meaningful life, meaningful activities and relationships, and addressing the underlying causes for problem behaviors.

Slide 8

The manner in which we approach others can have a significant impact on their feelings and behavior. If we are tense or anxious, the person we are interacting with is likely to become tense or anxious. Since tension or anxiety can serve as contributing events for problem behavior, we must try to ensure our actions do not create these feelings in others. On the other hand, if our actions con-

MODULE VI

tribute to positive emotions, these emotions can serve as contributing events for appropriate behavior.

Slide 9

Support Strategies

2. **Environmental Contributors to Problem Behaviors**

- Important to evaluate the environment

- **Look for things that might be contributing to, or triggering, problem behaviors**

NOTE:

Important to look at environment from the person's perspective.

Griffiths, Gardner, and Nugent, 1998

Before implementing treatment strategies for problem behavior, the places in which the behavior occurs should be assessed. When we evaluate the environment in which the problem behavior is occurring, we are looking for things that might be contributing to, or triggering, these difficulties. Features of the environment that may serve as triggers or contributing events include:

Noise
Uncomfortable temperatures
Poor lighting
Uncomfortable clothes
Lack of privacy, visual over-stimulation, limited space

It is important to look at the environment from the individual's perspective. For example, a room that seems perfectly quiet and calm, for one person, may be experienced as over-stimulating by a person with autism.

Slide 10

Exercise

Activity: *Consider environmental contributors and solutions for the following behaviors*

•Eduardo has been removing his clothes in the classroom. This only occurs in the winter months when he is often wearing sweaters.

•Laura will scream and bite her hand at the kitchen table during meal times.

•Angel bangs his head against the window on the school bus. Recently, the bus changed routes so this changed the order of his pick up and the location of his seat on the bus.

Slide 11

3. **Providing Choice and Self Determination**

    Guiding Principle: Choice has positive benefits

    • increases community integration

    • increases adaptive behavior

    • improves overall quality of life

    • decreases problem behavior

Providing individuals with choice and control over their lives is a founding principle in person-centered planning, self-determination, and many other positive initiatives undertaken by families, self-advocates, and professionals over the past ten to twenty years. The promotion of choice and control is based on

M
O
D
U
L
E

V
I

the belief that individuals prefer to have choices and that making choices for oneself has positive benefits.

Research on this topic suggests that when individuals with an intellectual/developmental disability have choice and control in their lives they experience increased community integration, as well as increases in adaptive behavior (Kern, et al., 1998). This makes a good deal of sense when we think about it. After all, if an individual has, for example, a choice in what he or she is going to eat for dinner, it seems logical he or she would be more interested in learning to prepare the meal.

Slide 12

The use of calming or relaxation techniques is an often-overlooked strategy in helping to prevent problem behavior. The teaching of calming strategies really serves one purpose. That purpose is to help the individual self-manage stress, tension, or anger, all of which may serve as contributing or triggering events for problem behavior. Relaxation strategies are also effective because they distract the person from the source of the stress and focus the person on an appropriate behavior. There are many types of relaxation, which are covered in Module VII, but we give the most common and simplest strategy here as an example.

Deep Breathing:

1. Sit or lie down
2. Breath in slowly through the nose and try to ensure the stomach rises
3. Slowly exhale while counting or saying "relax"
4. Repeat 10 times

Slide 13

Relaxation

Let's practice together
PMR: Progressive Muscle Relaxation

Sit in a relaxed position

Focus on yourself and on achieving relaxation in specific body muscles.

Tune out all other thoughts

Squeeze fists together tightly. Slowly count to five and release

Shrug your shoulders up to your ears for five seconds. Relax.

Arch your back off the floor for five seconds. Relax.

Squeeze legs tightly and slowly count to 5 and release

Repeat for other body parts that are tense

Avoid body parts that are sore of uncomfortable

Guide the participants in PMR, cautioning attendees to avoid sleep. Ask the attendees what their experiences were in practicing PMR.

MODULE VI

Slide 14

> # What do you find relaxing?
>
> **Activity: Think of an activity that you find relaxing:**
> •Playing an instrument? Listening to music? Attending concert?
> •Taking a walk or hiking?
> •Word puzzles or board games?
> •Dancing, aerobics, jogging or other exercise?
> •Watching TV? Going to the movies?
> •Cooking, reading, sewing, scrapbooking
>
> Using your interest and familiarity, design an activity for an individual or group in the setting where you work that promotes proactive relaxation opportunities. Build the most successful ideas into your regular routine!

Slide 15

> Support Strategies
>
> **5. Verbal Strategy**
> • Verbal techniques can help an individual feel acknowledged and supported
>
> • **Verbal techniques can be used by direct care staff as well as clinical staff**
>   a. **Validating**
>   b. **Exploring**
>   c. **Problem Solving**
>
> Sender Message
> Feedback
> Receiver

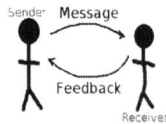

How we use our words can have a significant impact on whether an angry or agitated individual will engage in problem behavior. By using simple verbal strategies, we can communicate that we are sincerely interested in the person, are concerned about the person's problems, and are willing to help. When we communicate feelings such as these, we can often prevent problem behavior from occurring.

Exploring, validating, and problem solving can help develop a therapeutic relationship and thereby help prevent problem behavior.

Slide 16

Support Strategies

5. a) Validating

Validating involves confirming the person's emotions.

An example of this is shown in the following scenario:

Jack: "Everybody around here hates me!"

Staff: "It sounds as though you are pretty angry."

Hughes, 2006

In the example above the staff did not challenge Jack's feelings or beliefs by telling Jack everyone likes him. Rather, the staff validated Jack's feeling and attempted to encourage Jack to further explain what made him feel this way. Challenging Jack's feelings (e.g., "No, Jack, everybody likes you.") would probably have led to more frustration (contributing event) and increased the chances for problem behavior. Correcting peoples' perceptions can feel dismissive or like the staff does not really understand the issue.

The author most associated with this is Naomi Feil, who works primarily with persons experiencing dementia, but her strategies translate perfectly for persons with IDD and MI (Feil, 1993). She also encourages questioning the person and asking him/her to describe more of his/her feelings and thoughts as a means of de-escalation.

Slide 17

> Support Strategies
>
> 5. b) Validating & Exploring
>
> Validating and Exploring can be combined and involve encouraging the individual to further explain whatever it is the individual is trying to communicate
>
> An example of this is shown in the following scenario:
>
> Jack: "Everybody around here hates me!"
>
> Staff: "It sounds like you are pretty angry. Can you tell me what you are so mad about?"
>
> Hughes, 2004

Exploration provides an opportunity for the staff to be an active listener and for the client to have an opportunity to discuss issues and concerns. The combination of using both validating and exploring strategies can be effective techniques in helping individuals to decrease tension and stress. The staff must evaluate the person's readiness to move forward to exploring strategies. Delivering information before people are ready to move forward can be overwhelming and counterproductive.

Slide 18

Support Strategies

5. c) Problem Solving

- Identify the nature of the problem from the client's point of view.

- Explore alternative solutions to the problem

- Implement the best alternative solution

Problem solving can be a strategy used informally by DSP's or in a more formal way by clinicians. For DSP's problem solving approaches are appropriate for working with the client in his/her environment when the client is calm and ready to move forward. Staff must be cautious to avoid moving too quickly from validating to exploring and then problem-solving. This could be, for example, in a residential environment. It is a here and now "in-vivo" approach to problem solving. A problem solving approach can also be used by mental health clinicians in an office environment. This is different than an "in-vivo" approach as it requires a great deal more time and is significantly more methodical in its application.

Slide 19

> **Support Strategies**
>
> ### Exercise: Verbal Strategies
>
> You are working with a woman named Lorraine who believes that one of her staff or roommates steals her clothes from the laundry room. As a result she will no longer wash her clothes, wearing the same soiled outfits to work every day. When you approach Lorraine about this, she screams and yells about people stealing and not trusting anyone to help her.
>
> Activity: *consider the 3 verbal strategies reviewed on the prior slides to help Lorraine feel acknowledged and supported in reaching a productive and positive outcome.*

Slide 20

> **Effective Communication Strategies**
>
> There are certain communication techniques which can be very helpful in de-escalating situations. These include:
>
> 1. **Active Listening**
> 2. **Empathetic responses**
> 3. **Maintain a non-judgmental attitude**
>
> McGinley & Sweetland, 2011

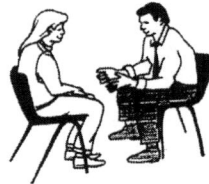

1. <u>Active Listening</u> -This involves reflecting back to the person what you have heard him or her say.

2. <u>Empathetic responses</u> - There is a difference between sympathy and em-

pathy. Giving a sympathetic response is a response reflecting your feelings. Empathy is the ability to understand another person's feelings and to understand how the person views a situation.

3. Maintain a non-judgmental attitude- This conveys an attitude that you accept the person and you are not critical. This does not mean that you are necessarily accepting the behavior, just understanding it is important to the person. It is important to maintain a calm, matter-of-fact, and neutral voice. Aggression leads to aggression, i.e., if care providers are verbally aggressive or hostile, it is more likely that the person will react in kind.

Slide 21

Effective Communication Strategies

4. **Recognize and avoid power struggles**

5. Watch your posture and body language

6. **Validate feelings**

7. Put the choices back to the person

4. Avoid power struggles- It is important in interacting with the people that you work with that you do not get into arguments with them. Avoid being confrontational and avoid arguing with them. Avoid trying to control things that are not essential for safety or structure.

5. Watch your posture and body language- Avoid any physical stance or posture that can be viewed as challenging.

6. Validate how they are feeling- You can validate the person's feelings without agreeing with the person.

7. <u>Put the choices back to the person-</u> If someone's behavior is escalating you can say, "You have a decision to make. You can hit someone or you can…" Put it back on the person and remind the person of the more productive and effective choices that can be made.

Slide 22

> Crisis Prevention and Planning
>
> **People who have a Dual Diagnosis are at risk of experiencing a crisis for a number of reasons:**
> - Medications/medical complications
> - **Changing life circumstances**
> - Inappropriate/inadequate supports
> - **Increase in mental health symptoms**
> - Substance abuse problems
> - **Behavioral phenotypes of genetic disorders**

A crisis is a serious deterioration of a person's ability to cope with every day life. It does not necessarily involve danger of serious physical harm to self or others but does require planning and support.

Due to the complex support needs of a person who has a dual diagnosis, frequent medical/mental health support is often needed. Knowing this in advance of the occurrence of a crisis allows for planning to be done to provide direction and intervention steps and strategies which can help minimize the duration and severity of the crisis for the person or possibly prevent the crisis completely. The intention of crisis planning is to reduce the risk of the crisis occurring and the risk to the person. Crisis management approaches can help a person avoid having to go to a crisis center, emergency room, hospital or have an encounter with the criminal justice system.

Slide 23

> Crisis Prevention and Planning
>
> **By addressing environmental, biological, psychological and social factors that may contribute to problem behavior, staff may be able to assist the person to cope, maintain control of his/her own behavior, and learn positive, productive ways that address the function of the behavior.**

Some of the prevention strategy considerations to be aware of for people who have a dual diagnosis:

- Maintain an appropriate activity/interest level for the person's needs.
- Know internal triggers related to past history, health, psychiatric conditions a person may experience, effects of medications, etc.
- Be aware of external environmental triggers – room temperature, noises, people, disorganization if they need things done in a certain way, disappointments, etc.
- Support the person to develop positive relationships.
- Reduce the stress around transitions.

Identifying the factors that contribute to problem behavior is a component of a Functional Assessment as discussed in Module II (Integrated Assessments).

MODULE VI

Slide 24

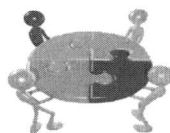

Crisis Prevention and Planning

Ensure the plan includes a description of what a crisis is for a specific person

Outline the appropriate actions to address the issues at the earliest possible stage of the crisis unfolding.

The plan should also include appropriate intervention strategies that are effective when dealing with problem behavior.

A Crisis Plan includes:
- A clear description of what constitutes a crisis for the person
- Clearly outlined actions to be taken and by whom at different identified points along the path of the crisis as it unfolds
- Contact information for resources/services/people who need to be contacted when a crisis occurs.

Slide 25

Crisis Management

Non-Verbal De-Escalation Strategies

1. Monitor your body position and body language

2. Avoid physically putting yourself in harm's way

3. Maintain a demeanor of calmness, neutrality, and confidence

McGillivray & Evans (used, 2001)

I. <u>Monitor your body position and body language </u>- Do not engage in any posturing that can be construed as aggressive or intimidating. For example, don't get in the person's space, point a finger at the person, or give body language cues that signal hostility.

2. <u>Avoid physically putting yourself in harm's way-</u> For example, avoid directly facing an agitated person and putting yourself directly in front of that person. This would make the front of your body fully vulnerable to getting hit. Keep a safe distance of at least 3-4 arm lengths away. This will decrease the likelihood of the person grabbing, punching, pulling, or lunging at you.

3. <u>Maintain a demeanor of calmness, neutrality, and confidence-</u> You want to present with a non-judgmental demeanor but one that indicates you are also attentive. If the person is feeling out-of-control, he or she needs to know that someone around him or her is going to take control if needed. This gives the person a sense of security.

Slide 26

1. Use a calm tone of voice- Avoid showing any strong emotional reaction to the person.

2. Use reflective listening- Reflect back the feelings you think you are hearing and seeing. For example, "I know that must have really upset you."

3. Avoid threatening punishment- You can remind the person of the possible consequences of his or her actions without threatening punishment. For example, you can say "Now remember, you are working toward that week-end pass."

4. Avoid power struggles- It is important the person feels his or her views are important and valid. Getting into a conversation about who is "right" can cause a power struggle, so avoid those conversations.

5. Do not ignore escalations of behaviors that could lead to severe behaviors- Intervene as early in the stages of escalation as possible

Slide 27

> Crisis Management
>
> **Verbal De-Escalation Strategies**
>
> 6. Change staffing if necessary
>
> **7. Affirm that you understand**
>
> 8. Change the subject if it appears to agitate the person more to talk about it (i.e., offer a drink of water, bring up an topic that interests him or her such as sporting event or TV program)
>
> McGowan & .... 22.

6. <u>Change staffing if necessary-</u> If the individual is very angry at you, it would not be helpful to continue to try and deal with that person. Have another staff take over. Otherwise the person is likely to continue staying agitated in your presence. Also, if you feel you can no longer deal with a person effectively on that shift because of your own emotional reactions, ask another staff to assist or take over. We are only human. Another staff can intervene to redirect the individual to another activity or let him or her vent appropriately.

7. <u>Affirm that you understand-</u> You do not need to communicate that you agree with the person's perspective, simply that you understand that whatever happened was upsetting from that person's perspective.

8. <u>Change the subject if it appears to agitate the person more to talk about it-</u> Help the individual focus on something else. If he or she keeps ruminating about the issue that caused the anger, the agitation will continue. An effective example is offering the person a drink of water or some other tangible item. It is both supportive for the person who is agitated and offers a distraction/change of topic from the subject which is causing the agitation.

Slide 28

> **Crisis Management**
>
> **Verbal De-Escalation Strategies**
>
> 9. Change aspects of the environment.
>
> 10. **Set limits by reminding the person of the choices and outcomes but do so in a firm, fair manner and with a non-emotional tone of voice.**
>
> 11. Remind the individual of the desirable consequences of choosing a positive behavior as opposed to a problem behavior. Then remind the persons of the undesirable consequences that can occur if he or she engages in the problem behavior.
>
> McGivery & Sweetland, 2011

9. <u>Change aspects of the environment-</u> For example, decrease stimulation in the environment in order to produce a more calming and peaceful environment. Simply turning off a TV or moving people out of the room can have a calming effect.

10. <u>Be limit setting by reminding the person of the rules but do so in a firm, fair manner and with a non-emotional tone of voice-</u> For example, if a client is yelling and screaming at another person in the living environment, the staff could inform the client that this behavior is not acceptable.

11. <u>Remind the individual of the desirable consequence if he/she chooses a more acceptable/appropriate behavior and the undesirable consequences that can occur if he or she engages in the behavior-</u> For example, a client is yelling and screaming in the home as mentioned above, and the person does not stop the behavior; the staff should remind the client that discontinuing the behavior will result in being able to go out as planned but the continuation of his behavior will result in the consequence of not going out with the other residents that evening (consequence articulated in the client's service plan). By leading with the desirable consequence, the staff is refocusing on the positive outcomes, which has greater potential to positively influence the choices the person makes.

Slide 29

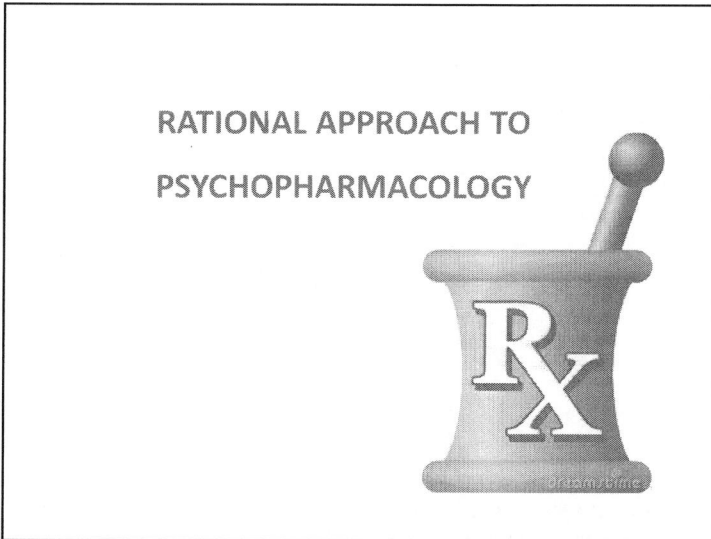

RATIONAL APPROACH TO

PSYCHOPHARMACOLOGY

Slide 30

MYTH: MEDICATION TREATMENT IS
USED TO CONTROL MALADAPTIVE
BEHAVIORS

<u>Premise</u>:
Medication-based therapies directly affect behavior.

<u>Reality:</u>
Behaviors such as self-injury and aggression are too nonspecific to be considered as direct targets for drug therapy.

<u>Treatment implications</u>:
The appropriate targets for medication therapy are the changes in neurophysiological function that mediate behavior associated with psychiatric disorders.

A rational approach to using medication is to target the underlying psychiatric disorder. For example, using an anti-depressant medication for persons who are diagnosed with major depression.

Another example is using a anti-psychotic medication for persons who are diagnosed with schizophrenia.

A third example is using an anti-anxiety medication for people who are diagnosed with an anxiety disorder.

The take home message is to use medication treatment associated with a specific psychiatric disorder.

Slide 31

Medication Treatment

Pharmacotherapy is therapeutic and may be the first choice treatment for some psychiatric disorders:

• Major depression

• Mania states

• Schizophrenia

Medication treatment should be diagnostically related to a DSM 5 diagnostic and treatment guideline or the DM-ID.

Medication treatment is often used as the first choice of treatment for mental health issues and/or problem behavior. This is the case when medication treatment is needed to stabilize the individual's mental health or assist to calm someone who is physically and emotionally struggling for control. Once the person has been reasonably stabilized, then other supportive approaches can be applied.

Please note that referral for medication therapy can often take a significant period of time. Concurrent positive supports, environmental adaptation, when possible, and supportive responses by caregivers are necessary while awaiting consultation and for mediation therapy to reach efficacy levels.

Psychotropic medication use can be therapeutic for long term stabilization of serious mental illness and should be considered as part of a comprehensive treatment plan when appropriate.

Slide 32

> # Putting it all together
>
> Activity: Develop a blueprint wellness plan for someone you support. Consider the support strategies reviewed in this chapter that would apply to him/her.
>
> Tips
> - Identity the person's strengths and interests
> - Consider the person's diagnosis and mental health needs
> - Promote relaxation opportunities
> - Anticipate challenges and be prepared with de-escalation and validation strategies
> - Build in ways to help the person feel good about him/herself and develop positive identify
> - Monitor behavior and medication information

References: Module VI

Carr, J.E, Sidener, T.M. (2002). On the relation between applied behavior analysis and positive behavioral support. *The Behavior Analyst, 25*, 245–253.

Feil, N. (1993). *The validation breakthrough: Simple techniques for communicating with people with Alzheimer's-type dementia.* Baltimore, MD: Health Professions Press.

Griffiths, D., Gardner, W.I., & Nugent, J. (1998). Behavioral supports: individual centered interventions: A multi-modal functional approach. *Journal of Intellectual Disability Research, 44*(2), 182-184.

Hughes, E.E. (2006). The *dual diagnosis primer: A training manual for family members, case managers, advocates, guardians and direct support professionals.* Kingston, N.Y.: NADD Press.

Kern, L., Vorndran, M., Hilt, A., Ringhahl, J., Adelman, B., & Dunlap, G. (1998). Choice as an intervention to improve behavior. *A Review of the Literature Journal of Behavioral Education, 8*(2), 151-169.

McGilvery, S. & Sweetland, D. (2011). *Intellectual disability and mental health: A training manual in dual diagnosis.* Kingston, N. Y.: NADD Press.

Adapting Therapy for People with IDD

Slide 1

> ### Module VII
>
> #### Adapting Therapy for
> #### People with IDD

Slide 2

> This module introduces concepts in Adapting Therapy to make it more useful for persons with IDD.
>
> This modules discusses concepts in mental wellness.

Slide 3

> # Learning Objectives
>
> - **List reasons why people with IDD seek therapy**
> - **List ways to make therapy more accessible to people with IDD**
> - **Describe the principles and benefits of DBT, CBT and Individual /Group Therapy**
> - **Describe how trauma effects people with IDD**
> - **Describe the trauma treatment strategies and adaptations for IDD**
> - **Describe how to support a person in positive Identity Development**

Slide 4

> **Adapted Therapies**
>
> **Myth:** Persons with IDD are not appropriate for psychotherapy
>
> **Premise:** Impairments in cognitive abilities and language skills make psychotherapy ineffective.
>
> **Reality:** Level of intelligence is not a sole indicator for appropriateness of therapy.
>
> **Treatment Applications:** Psychotherapy approaches need to be adapted to the expressive and receptive language skills of the person.
>
> Benson 2013

There is an increasing acceptance of the use of psychotherapy for people with IDD. The issue is no longer whether people with IDD are entitled to psycho-therapy or can benefit from it, but how the psychotherapy techniques can be adapted to meet the needs of people who have limitations in expressive and receptive language skills.

Slide 5

Adapted Therapies

- Relationship between a client and a therapist/counselor

- **Engaged in a therapeutic relationship**

- To achieve a change in emotions, thoughts or behavior

The purpose of psychotherapy or counseling is no different than the purpose used for the general population. How we define psychotherapy/counseling is also the same.

Slide 6

Similarities Between Children without IDD And Adults with IDD

Without IDD	With IDD
6-7 Years Old	6-7 Years Old Cognitive Level Mild IDD Borderline IDD

Both usually dependent on others

Both tend to be in supervised settings

Both have cognitive limitations in terms of:
    Problem solving
    Impulse control
    Concrete thought

Research has demonstrated that there are general similarities between life issues faced by children without IDD and adults with mild level IDD. Children are referred for therapy when issues arise, but adults with IDD who have similar issues are generally not considered candidates for therapy.

Slide 7

> **Similarities Between Children without IDD And Adults with IDD**
>
> - **Both struggle with issues of:**
>   **Independence**
>   **Peer group**
>   **Identity choices**
>   **Vocational**
>   **Sexual identity**
>   **Authority issues**
>
> - **Both referred to therapy by others**
>
> Prout & Strohmer, 1994

There is a striking similarity in the treatment issues for adolescents without IDD and adults with mild level of IDD. One needs to consider the cognitive developmental level of the person with mild levels of IDD. Despite the chronological age of the adult with mild level IDD, he/she is likely to have similar treatment issues as adolescents without IDD.

If an adolescent is having emotional issues, he/she may be recommended for psychotherapy. Likewise, we should think about psychotherapy for adults with IDD who also struggle with emotional issues.

Slide 8

Why People with and without IDD Seek Therapy	
Interpersonal Concerns	22%
General Psychological Functioning	18%
Work	12%
Sexuality	6%
Family	5%
Residential Living & Adjustment	5%
Behavior	4%
Financial & Material Resources	4%
Accepting & Coping with Disability	4%
Dealing with Authority Figures	4%
Other	16%

Willner, Strohmer & Prout, 19??

The reasons people with IDD seek support/therapy can be as varied as the reasons for which a neuro-typical person engages in therapy.

Slide 9

Adapted Therapies

Cognitive Load of Therapy and Intervention

Cognitive Load refers to the amount of information and interactions processed simultaneously (or) thinking and reasoning required for people to build on what they already understand.

- Many of the typical ways we provide therapy are complex and require significant cognitive functioning to work
- Typical practices may not work for a person with IDD.

Many different types of therapy have been found to be effective in treating people with IDD. Treatment providers need a strategy for adaptation so language, goals, strategies, and tasks can be adapted to the intellectual/developmental abilities of the client.

Slide 10

> **Adapted Therapies**
>
> **Many typical therapy sessions start with this question:** "Have you been feeling better since last time I saw you?"
>
> - Must remember feelings from last visit
> - Must know current feelings
> - Must be able to compare
> - Must know what the therapist is really asking
> - Must be able to inductively reason
>
> And so on and so on...

Traditional, non-adapted therapy models require significant memory retention and self-awareness that may exceed the cognitive ability of person who has a dual diagnosis (questions that require high cognitive load to process and respond). Morasky (2007) also suggests that to help figure out what needs to be adapted, the therapist must first ask what makes the intellectual activity difficult for the person. This is the area for which adaptation is required.

Slide 11

There are therapies that have been formally adapted for use with people with a dual diagnosis: DBT (dialectic behavior therapy), some trauma specific therapies, and CBT (cognitive behavior therapy).

Slide 12

Principles of achieving a therapeutic relationship are relevant to a psychotherapist. Also, most of these principles are relevant to other care providers who are involved in support of an individual who has IDD.

Empathetic understanding – Trying to understand the "inner world" of the individual. What would it be like to be in his/her shoes?

Respect and acceptance of the client – This is a fundamental principle that is essential in developing a therapeutic relationship. It is analogous to Carl Rogers' concept of "unconditional regard."

Concreteness – Using language that is understood by the person with IDD. Avoid analogies and use language appropriate to the language skills of the client.

Therapeutic genuineness – This implies being yourself in a real and authentic way.

Accept the client's life circumstances – Many of the individuals we serve have horrendous backgrounds. Regardless of the nature or extent of "background baggage" he/she carries, it is important that we accept the individual. The life circumstances of the individuals we serve should not have a negative influence on how we value the individual.

Slide 13

Confidentiality

- Nothing discussed in therapy will be released without the person's permission

- With the client's permission, the therapist will work collaboratively other care providers

Confidentiality traditionally means that there is an expectation of both the therapist and the client that what happens between them is private in that the information revealed during their interactions will not be divulged to others under ordinary circumstances. "What is said in the session, stays in the session."

However, when conducting therapy with a person who has IDD/MI it is important for the therapist to communicate with family members and other care providers involved in the person's life. This communication is done only after the client has given both verbal and written permission. If the client is under age 18 or has a legal guardian, the permission may also involve the parent or legal guardian.

In essence, the therapist should not work in isolation. Rather, the therapist works, in a conceptual way, as part of the person's treatment or habilitative team. The communication from the therapist should be around conceptual issues and not details of what was discussed in therapy.

Slide 14

Therapy can be an intellectually challenging activity. Much of the therapy that exists presumes quite a lot of cognitive activity and ability for the person. These are some of the most significant ones.

MODULE VII

Slide 15

Providing therapy for people with a dual diagnosis is not significantly different than providing therapy for people in the general population. The principles of therapy remain the same, but the approach to therapy is modified. Approaches to therapy are adapted according to the expressive and receptive language skills of the individual.

The model described here is appropriate for persons who have IDD co-occurring with MI. This model can be used for either short term or long term therapy. It is rather simplistic but contains the essential components needed to realize positive outcomes.

Slide 16

Active Listening – It is important for the therapist to demonstrate active listening skills. Good eye contact and body posture are two ways in which we can communicate to the individual our interest. With permission from the client, a tap on the shoulder, at the beginning of the session can indicate a caring message, which can set the positive tone and demonstrate interest in the client.

MODULE VII

Slide 17

Reflect – Using a reflective technique can be very valuable in "checking out" whether the client and clinician understood that which is being communicated. The client statements are re-stated or re-phrased to the client, so as to emphasize their emotional significance.

Slide 18

Probe – It is generally useful for the therapist to take an active role in the therapy process. At times it may be difficult for a person with IDD to have a "back and forth conversation" in the absence of the therapist taking an active role. It is difficult for individuals with IDD to answer questions that begin with "why." This is because "why" questions generally require the client to think abstractly. Questions should be relevant to the person's language skills. Asking an individual to describe a situation can be a useful method of probing.

Slide 19

Therapy Model

Support

- **Supportive statements indicate understanding**

- **Express that you care**

- **Acknowledge having been in a similar situation**

Support – Providing support during the course of the therapy process is important. It acknowledges the value of the individual and conveys an expression of concern and caring. It can normalize the individual's feelings and responses.

Slide 20

Exercise

Pair up and practice active listening. Each person gets to be the speaker and the listener. Make sure to use all of the active listening strategies described on the previous slides.

Slide 21

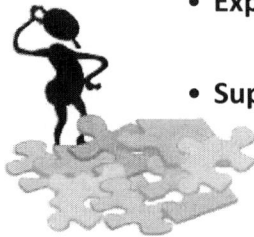

Therapy Model

Facilitate problem solving

- **Explore alternative options**

- **Support acceptable solutions**

Facilitate Problem Solving – Facilitating problem solving can be considered the "meat & potato" of therapy. Once the problem has been clearly identified, the client can explore two or three alternative options to address the problem. It can be useful to have the problem written on a piece of paper along with the alternative solutions to the problem. Then, the client and therapist can analyze the alternative solutions by identifying the pros and cons of each alternative solution. This to can be written on paper as a visual. Lastly, an acceptable alternative option can be selected and supported by both the client and therapist.

The therapist can give the client a "homework assignment" related to the problem and solution. This is a concrete tool to help the client stay on track and maintain continuity from one session to another. The therapist can also develop a self monitoring tool to enable the client to self monitor work conducted outside the therapy session and to measure progress.

Slide 22

Therapy Model

Evaluate outcome

- **Was outcome acceptable?**
- **Was it positive?**
- **What was learned?**

Evaluate Outcome – There are several ways in which the outcome of therapy can be evaluated. One way is for the client to use a self monitoring tool to measure progress. Another way to evaluate is through the client's self report of progress, which can be obtained during the therapy session. A third way is to obtain information from parents and other care providers regarding the individual's change in behavior as it relates to the therapeutic goal.

Slide 23

Slides 11-13 identify best practices in how to adapt therapy for persons with IDD, using a strength-based model. The following slides show ways do to that specifically.

Slide 24

Slide 25

> **Best Practice**
>
> ### ...Continued
>
> 3. Positive behavior supports
>
> a. Management of problem behavior relies upon identifying reasons for problem behavior
>
> b. Look into different areas of life in terms of understanding problem behaviors
>
> c. Intervention targets strength based planning, support
>
> d. Identification, teaching and wellness approaches
>
> Bauer & Blumberg, 2008

The therapies listed in the past three slides above share commonalities:
* Strength-based support.
* Meet a person where he or she is.
* Rather than focusing on something going away, focus on adding something.

Slide 26

> **Best Practice**
>
> ### 4. Adapting Instruction in General
>
> * Size
> * Time
> * Level of Support
> * Input
> * Difficulty
>
> * Output
> * Participation
> * Alternate
> * Substitute Curriculum
>
> Deschenes, Ebeling, & Sprague, 1994

Adaptations to all these components of therapy are required to make it accessible to people who have intellectual and cognitive challenges. Although there are a number of issues that must be addressed when providing psychotherapy to individuals with intellectual disabilities and mental illnesses, many psychotherapeutic techniques are effective if they are suitably modified.

Slide 27

Adaptations

Size

Adapt the number of items that the person is expected to learn or complete.

General example: If person is to know the fifty states, have persons only be responsible for remembering a certain number at a time. This would be dependent on the person's level of disability.

Therapeutic Example: In doing the "Three Good Things" intervention from Positive Psychology, the client is asked to only generate "One Good Thing."

Doycrene:, Eveling, & Spragon, 1994

Positive psychotherapy

Seligman and colleagues at the University of Pennsylvania developed positive psychotherapy as a way to treat depression by building positive emotions, character strengths, and sense of meaning, not just by reducing negative symptoms such as sadness. This therapy uses a combination of 12 exercises that can be practiced individually or in groups. Some key themes of all the different strategies include: (a) a focus on identifying the skills and interests that the person has, (b) identifying resources that the person can use, (c) working with individual to identify specific support needs, and (d) arranging support to address those needs.

Three good things. The concept involves daily listing three good things that happened.   for a person who has a dual diagnosis, as recommended above, they may be request to identify one item in a day. This adaptation takes into consideration difficulties with memory retention and recall as well as focus on multiple concepts simultaneously.

Slide 28

Adaptations

Time

Adapt the time allotted and allowed for learning, task completion, or testing.

For example: Allow person additional time to complete timed assignments. However, if the total project is due by a particular time, have the person complete each portion of the project over various intervals with the required finished project due at a later time.

Therapeutic Example: The client is allowed extra time to answer questions.

This adaptation takes into consideration challenges a person may have related to the level of cognitive impairment including working memory and executive functioning related skill deficits. Many persons with ASDs may respond more slowly to information presented auditorially, so additional time for responding can be offered.

Slide 29

> ### Level of Support
> Adaptations
>
> **Increase the amount of personal assistance with a specific person.**
>
> **For example:** Allow for peer teaching. Pair the slower persons with the more advanced persons in order to provide support.
>
> **Therapeutic Example:** In Narrative Therapy, the client is given additional prompting and reminders.

In Narrative Therapy, the process of externalization allows people to consider their relationships with problems, thus the narrative motto: "The person is not the problem, the problem is the problem." So-called strengths or positive attributes are also externalized. When adapting this for a client with an intellectual or cognitive impairment, the therapist will participate more in prompting the client to develop a more comprehensive narrative about the problem to help focus the effects on the person's life and investigate problem solving options. (White &Epston, 1990). This adaptation considers and makes compensation for impairments in executive functioning related to working memory and includes past knowledge into current discussions. It also considers adaptation for delays in processing verbal information and forming a response – receptive and expressive language deficits.

Slide 30

Adaptations

Input

Adapt the way instruction is delivered to the person.

For example: Provide persons with a audio and/or video tape of the lesson. Allow for field trips, guest speakers, peer teaching, computer support, video productions.

Therapeutic Example: Concrete objects can be used in Cognitive Behavior Therapy.

If cognitive behavior therapy is used a part of a stress management or anxiety intervention, objects can be used to represent the stress management practice. For example a feather can be used to illustrate blowing in and blowing out.

Slide 31

Adaptations

Difficulty

Reduce the difficult of the Task

For example: Allow the person to be creative providing that task is completed according to instructor's specifications. For example the person may draw a picture of the assignment, do an interview, etc. depending on subject. Allow the person to come up with the idea. Accept any reasonable modifications.

Therapeutic Example: Allow the person to use a variety of different relaxation responses.

Traditional and non-traditional relaxation techniques can be effective for people with IDD with appropriate adaptation as needed.

* Progressive muscle relaxation (PMR) involves tensing and relaxing muscle groups
* Visualisation or guided imagery involves asking an individual to imagine, for example, a peaceful scene
* Focussed breathing - increasing one's awareness and control of breathing patterns.
* Autogenics - listening to positive self-statements and affirmations, such as "my breathing is smooth and rhythmical" and "I am in control".
* Snoezelen multisensory environments
* Ti Chi, Yoga, Meditation, aromatherapy, music,
* Behavioral Relaxation Training involves modeling both relaxed and non-relaxed behaviors across 10 areas of the body (head, mouth, hands, feet, body, breathing, throat, eyes, shoulders, and vocalizations) with imitation by the client. After observing postures, the person is encouraged to imitate the appropriate behaviors. Rather than rely on self-reporting to gauge anxiety reduction, BRT uses an assessment scale for external cues that can be observed and scored by the clinician. (Poppen, 1998)

Slide 32

Adaptations

Output

Adapt how the person can respond to instruction.

For example: Allow persons to draw pictures, write an essay, complete specific computer software program relating to lesson.

Therapeutic Example: Allow the client to draw responses or use a communication device to answer questions. A menu board of responses offers a choice of answers, reducing the need for crude recall.

Rather than focusing solely on verbal responding, allow the individual to use augmentative or alternative forms of communication to answer questions.

Slide 33

> **Adaptations**
>
> ### Participation
>
> **Adapt the extent to which a person is actively involved in the task.**
>
> **For example:** Tailor the person's participation in a task to his or her abilities, whether intellectual or physical.
>
> **Therapeutic Example:** Adapt Wellness Interventions, such as the promotion of experienced creativity, to include Partial Participation.

For art therapy, the individual can partially participate in the creation of art, directing the art therapist to paint certain things.

Slide 34

> **Adaptations**
>
> ### Alternate
>
> **Adapt the goals or outcome expectations while using the same materials.**
>
> **For example:** In a writing assignment, alter the expectations for a disabled person who takes longer to write a paragraph.
>
> **Therapeutic Example:** Allow them to dictate a Gratitude Letter as opposed to writing it themselves.

A gratitude letter is a suggested activity within the Positive Psychology frame-

MODULE VII

work. The concept involves writing a letter to someone explaining why you feel grateful for something they've done or said. Read the letter to the recipient, either in person or over the phone.

For a person with IDD this method can be adapted by limiting the number of items, the method by which the letter is created (a dictated letter, visual story board).

The adaptation is consistent with the goal and process of the gratitude letter, but considers adaptations for a person who may not have well developed literacy skills, the ability to keep track of more than one thing at a time,

Slide 35

Adaptations

Substitute Curriculum

Provide different instruction and materials to meet a person's individual goals.

For example: Instead of discussing the reasons for the civil war, have the disabled person work on a puzzle showing the Union and Confederate states.

Therapeutic Example: Teach coping instruction using simpler, less abstract example.

Adaptive functioning challenges can include difficulty with

- generalizing,
- Abstract thinking
- Problem solving

The individual can be guided in using simple methods for coping, such as power walking while the therapist models long breaths, as opposed to a complex systems of teaching coping.

Slide 36

> # Exercise
>
> **Get in small groups of 3-4. If you were going to teach a person with IDD to make a paper airplane, consider how to use each of the different adaptations from slide 26 to simplify the instruction.**

You are welcome to use your own example. If any attendees do not know how to make a paper airplane, you can show them. There is no single right way to make a paper airplane.

Slide 37

> **Psychological Interventions**
>
> **Recommendations Specific for Therapy for Persons with IDD**
>
> - **Morasky (2007) has provided an excellent description of strategies for adapting psychological intervention for persons with IDD, including modifying speed, number, abstraction, and complexity.**
>
>   – **Morasky, R. (2007). Making counseling/therapy intellectually attainable. *The NADD Bulletin, 10*, pp. 58-62.**

Slide 38

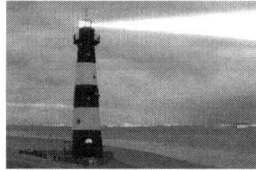

Psychological Interventions

Guiding Principles:

- Use language that promotes hope

- Raise expectations of what people are capable of accomplishing

- Stay focused on strengths

Guiding Principles - There are guiding principles for promoting mental wellness which can be used by staff at all levels. These principles come from the recovery model employed in the mental health field. The focus is strength-based and with an emphasis on success.

Slide 39

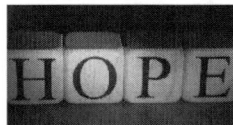

Psychological Interventions

- Build everyone's hope
- Instill a source of hope whenever possible
- Feeling a sense of hope for the future can be transformative

HOPE

Guiding Principles – The recovery model embraces the concept of hope. The role of the therapist, therefore, is to instill hope in the client. This is particularly poignant with individuals who have a dual diagnosis because they often have histories of abuse, neglect, and despair.

Slide 40

Guiding Principles – Celebrating accomplishments can be done in incremental ways. It is a way to express support for the individual. Celebrating accomplishments can be expressed when a client has acted in some positive manner. Frequent expression of accomplishments represents value for the individual and hope for the future.

Slide 41

Trauma Informed Intervention

Trauma

- **Trauma is the emotional response to a terrible event like an accident, rape or natural disaster.**
- **Immediately after the event, shock and denial are typical.**
- **Longer term reactions include unpredictable emotions, flashbacks, strained relationships and even physical symptoms like headaches or nausea (APA, 2013).**

Slide 42

Trauma Informed Intervention

A major trauma could be

- **Sexual Assault/Physical Assault**
- **Natural or manmade disasters**
- **Catastrophic illness**
- **Loss of a loved one**
- **Humiliation**
- **Bullying**
- **Deprivation and powerlessness to act on one's own behalf**

Not all trauma results in lasting problems for a person. Whether or not the trauma leads to longer term issues and lasting stress depends on
- Duration
- Intensity of stressor

- Time of day
- Warning/ no warning
- Intentionality/preventability
- Scope/numbers affected
- Support system during and after traumatic event(s).
- Previous history of traumas/stressors/abuse
- History or family history of mental illnesses
- Inherent resilience/vulnerability
- Substance abuse
- Difficult relationships/poor attachment to others. This is especially true if the trauma has been caused by another person or people.

Slide 43

Trauma Informed Intervention

Trauma

People with intellectual/developmental disabilities are at greater risk for being victimized or abused.

Some experts believe as many as 90% of people with intellectual disabilities have some level of traumatic stress. Sobsey (1994) reports that people with disabilities are twice as likely to experience abuse.

People with intellectual/developmental disabilities are also at great risk of experiencing longer term trauma due to the build up of every day stresses and losses which can be unique to their experiences.
- Feeling different
- Not being accepted
- Not being able to do what others do
- Moving to a new home or significant change at home
- Knowing that one has a disability and is "different" than others
- Not being listened to
- Being misunderstood

MODULE VII

- Failing at a task
- Getting confused and overwhelmed

(Adler-Tapia & Settle, 2009)

Slide 44

<table>
<tr><td>

Trauma Informed Intervention

People with IDD often manifest PTSD differently than what is typically recognized as PTSD in the DSM – V

Some individuals may have flashbacks, but are not able to communicate that experience. What they do communicate, rather, may be misunderstood as a psychotic disorder.

</td></tr>
</table>

One of the challenges is identifying that a traumatic event has even happened for a learning disabled individual, especially for those without well developed communication skills and when the event has happened long in the past, since some of the events most likely to cause PTSD, such as sexual abuse, occur without witnesses.

The general under-diagnosis of PTSD amongst people who have IDD leads to a large portion those with PTSD never receive treatment. One study of people who have IDD and PTSD as a result of experienced sexual abuse found that only 39% of victims received treatment from a therapist. (Sequeira, Howlin, & Hollins, 2003)

Slide 45

Simple and Complex PTSD

Big T traumas:
> *simple post-traumatic stress* resulting from a one-time incident — such as a rape ,violent assault, injury

Little t Traumas:
> *complex post-traumatic stress* is a complex set of responses that follows chronic, multiple, and/or ongoing traumatic events such as taunting, teasing, tormenting, prolonged abuse

---

Complex PTSD is a result of prolonged and repeated trauma occurs in situations where a person is captive, unable to flee, or is under the control of the perpetrator (Herman, 1992).

Cognitive behavioral therapy (CBT) has yielded positive results amongst individuals with learning disability and PTSD just as it has in the general population. An adapted CBT therapy developed a modified self report scale from 0 to 10 rather than 0 to 100; allowing the victim to use the past tense when relating the traumatic event (rather than using the present tense to explain the story as if it were occurring presently); and allowing a therapist to attend with the victim at the site of the original traumatic event because the person may not be sufficiently independent to do so on his/her own.

Francine Shapiro (2012) the founder of EMDR, asserts that small but traumatic events can accumulate to have a similar traumatic effect on an individual.

MODULE VII

Slide 46

> **Trauma Informed Intervention**
>
> ### Trauma Informed Intervention
> - Positive Identity Development
> - DBT – Dialectical Behavior Therapy
>   - Supportive Counseling
>   - Group Therapy
> - TF-CBT
> - EMDR
> - Individual Psychotherapy

There are a wide variety of different intervention packages for trauma treatment for persons with IDD that have an evidence base to support effectiveness. Each of these will be discussed in order.

Slide 47

> **Positive Identity Development**
>
> **Positive Identity Development**
>
> The presence of an intellectual/developmental disability impacts exposure to new experiences and the person's understanding and integration of those experiences.
>
> This requires the organization and delivery of identity-related supports and counseling for persons with IDD across the lifespan.

Identity forms through the accumulation of experience and the integration of experiences and interpretations of experience.

These experiences begin in infancy when children begin to recognize themselves. Since it is likely that persons with IDD will move through stages of identity development at a slower or different rate from persons in the general population.

A critical role for care providers and families exists in the need to support persons with IDD in the development of a healthy, accurate self-identity.

Slide 48

Positive Identity Development

Many people with an IDD have a largely negative sense of identity which is constituted of all the good things the person is not. Specific therapeutic approaches can help to create a more positive sense of identity.

MODULE VII

Slide 49

Positive Identity Development

"The therapist facilitates the discovery of self and then helps to strengthen and reinforce that sense of self from session to session."

Karen Harvey, 2009

Harvey, 2007

Slide 50

EMDR

Eye Movement Desensitization and Reprocessing (EMDR)

First developed by Francine Shapiro upon noticing that certain eye movements reduced the intensity of disturbing thought.

EMDR uses a person's own rapid, rhythmic eye movements.

Treatment consists of 8 phases with precise intentions.

Shapiro, 2012

EMDR is now recommended as an effective treatment for trauma in the *Practice Guidelines* of the American Psychiatric Association.

EMDR integrates elements from both psychological theories (e.g. affect, attachment, behavior, bioinformational processing, cognitive, humanistic, family systems, psychodynamic and somatic) and psychotherapies (e.g., body-based, cognitive-behavioral, interpersonal, person-centered, and psychodynamic) into a standardized set of procedures and clinical protocols.

Slide 51

Dialectical Behavior Therapy

Dialectical Behavior Therapy (DBT)

DBT is a comprehensive treatment program addressing deficits in emotion regulation, distress tolerance, and interpersonal relationships accomplished through:

- individual psychotherapy,
- skills training groups, and
- supervision/case consultation groups

Linehan, 1993a, 1993b

DBT was originally developed by Marsha Linehan (1993a; 1993b) for the treatment of individuals diagnosed with borderline personality disorder.

It is now best described as being designed for the severe and chronic, multi-diagnostic, difficult to treat client. DBT has been adapted to persons with IDD by Charlton and colleagues (Chalton, 2006; Charlton & Dykstra, 2011).

MODULE VII

Slide 52

> Dialectical Behavior Therapy
>
> ### Using DBT, therapists have five main tasks:
>
> - expand client capabilities,
> - motivate the client to engage in new behaviors,
> - generalize the use of the new behaviors,
> - establish a treatment environment that reinforces progress, and
> - maintain capable and motivated therapists
>
> Linehan, 2003

DBT (dialectic behavior therapy) for trauma focuses on mindfulness, emotional regulation, distress tolerance, and interpersonal effectiveness. The Skills System is an adaptation of Linehan's model and focuses on the four skills above. It can be taught without the whole DBT program. (Brown, 2011; Charlton, 2006)

Slide 53

> Therapeutic Effects Of Group Therapy
>
> ### 13 Benefits
>
> 1. Fosters meaningful relationships
>
> 2. Increases relationship skills
>
> 3. Promotes problem solving skills
>
> 4. Enables learning through observation
>
> Based on Yalom-etc., 2 05

Groups are a good forum for psycho-education.

Slide 54

Therapeutic Effects Of Group Therapy
13 Benefits

5. Helps decrease feelings of: inadequacy, isolation and defeat

6. Promotes peer support

7. Fosters a sense of security

8. Promotes group cohesiveness

9. Establishes sense of trust

Group therapy is It is effective for teaching coping skills, and group members can reinforce the work by sharing what they find helpful.

It helps break down the isolation.

MODULE VII

Slide 55

> **Therapeutic Effects Of Group Therapy**
>
> ### 13 Benefits
>
> 10. Promotes sense of belonging – shared experiences
>
> 11. Instills sense of hope - optimism
>
> 12. Facilitates altruism – helping others
>
> 13. Promotes self understanding

Group therapy helps normalize people's experience when others share their struggle.

Slide 56

> Cognitive Behavior Therapy
>
> **Cognitive Behavioral Therapy (CBT)**
>
> CBT is effective in helping clients improve functioning and in identifying the beliefs, feelings, and behaviors associated with the trauma responses.
>
> Overall functioning is improved through skills development and more adaptive cognitive appraisals of events that trigger intense responses.
>
> CBT teaches people to monitor thoughts and change thought patterns leading to problems. There is a strong evidence base showing utility for persons with IDD if proper adaptation is made (Gaus, 2007).

CBT is "problem focused" (undertaken for specific problems) and "action ori-

MODULE VII

ented" (therapist tries to assist the client in selecting specific strategies to help address those problems). Strategies may be presented in a variety of concrete media. For example, a client who is working on impulsive behavior may carry a picture of traffic lights representing "Stop. Think. Go" to prompt them to process emotions and thoughts before taking action.

Adaptations in CBT need to include consideration to:
Meaningfully include past knowledge in current discussions
Ability to evaluate ideas and reflect on actions taken
Have insight into and ability to express thoughts and feelings
Delays in processing verbal information and forming a response – receptive and expressive language deficits

Slide 57

Individual Psychotherapy

Individual Psychotherapy

Individual psychotherapy aims to increase the person's overall well being.

It is most effective when the therapist adapts the model to consider the cognitive ability of the person with intellectual/developmental disability.

Hollins & Sinason, 2000

Psychotherapy has been observed to be most effective when clinicians adapt standard technique to the patient's cognitive level,
being directive in approach,
being flexible during therapy,
engaging significant others in the therapeutic process,
carefully managing transference and countertransference issues, and
directly addressing the issue of cognitive challenges as a disability

Slide 58

Adapted Therapies

When implementing adapted therapies with people who have IDD, remember to :

- Slow down your speech
- Use language that is comprehensible to the person
- Present information one item at a time using different methods (visual, auditory)
- Take frequent pauses during the session to check comprehension
- Use multisensory input

Continued....

These are dimensions we specifically recommend for adapting therapy. Each of these should be considered for each person whom you support. You may not use all of them, but they all may be of value.

Slide 59

Adapted Therapies

Continued....

- Make specific suggestions for change
- Allow time to practice new skills
- Use more repetition
- Do not assume that information will generalize to new situations and spend more time working on generalization
- Do not assume the information is too complex for the person to understand

Your choice of which of these to use will be based on the learning style of the person, the type of therapy, and your specific aims.

Slide 60

Adapted Therapy

"Contracting"

Contracting is an informal counseling tool which outlines the understanding of both the client and the therapist about the process and expectations. It basically means, "We are on the same page about how this is going to go. "

Considerations for inclusion in the contract:
- Ask for permission to interrupt,
- Avoid using inappropriate language
- Types of tips people who have IDD will find useful regarding the therapy process.

Contracting is an agreement set up in therapy that helps a person understand what to expect and helps him or her to feel comfortable and safe. It can include information about confidentially, the length of the session, the topics that will be discussed and other things that are important to the client. The contract helps create structure and boundaries. This is particularly helpful for a person with IDD who may need reminders about the goals and expectations of the session.

MODULE VII

Slide 61

By adapting empirically validated psychotherapy techniques and treatments, a clinician can provide effective therapy for people with an IDD and MI.

With some consideration to cognitive abilities, including expressive and receptive language, psychotherapy techniques can be effectively adapted to meet the needs of people who have an IDD and an MI.

References: Module VII

Adler-Tapia, R.L., & Settle, C.S (2009, March). EMDR with children: The full works. *Counseling Children and Young People* [a divisional journal of the British Association for Counselling and Psychotherapy], 12-15.

American Psychiatric Association. (2013). Recovering emotionally from disaster. Retrieved February 2015 from http://www.apa.org/topics/trauma/index.aspx.

Baker, D.J, & Blumberg, E. (2008). The intersection of best practice in dual diagnosis and positive psychology. *NADD Bulletin.* 11(1), 10-13.

Brown, J. (2011). *The skills system instructor's guide: An emotion-regulation skills curriculum for all learning abilities.* Bloomington, IN: iUniverse.

Charlton, M. (2006). Dialectical behavior therapy for children with developmental disabilities. *NADD Bulletin,* 9(5): 90-97.

Charlton, M., & Dykstra, E.J. (2011). Dialectical behaviour therapy for special populations: treatment with adolescents and their caregivers. *Advances in Mental Health and Intellectual Disabilities.* 5(5), 6–14.

Charlton, M., & Tallant, B. (2003). Trauma treatment with clients who have dual diagnoses: Developmental disabilities and mental illness. *National Association for the Dually Diagnosed Annual Conference Proceedings.* Kingston, NY: NADD Press.

Deschenes, C., Ebeling, D., & Sprague, J. (1994). *Adapting curriculum and instruction in inclusive classrooms: A teacher's desk reference.* Bloomington, IN: University of Indiana - Institute for the Study of Developmental Disabilities.

Fletcher, R.J. (Ed.). (2011). *Psychotherapy for individuals with intellectual disability.* Kingston, NY: NADD Press.

Gaus, V.L. (2007). *Cognitive behavioral therapy for adult Asperger syndrome.* New York : Guilford Press.

Harvey, K. (2009). *Positive identity development: An alternative treatment approach for individuals with mild and moderate intellectual disabilities.* Kingston, NY: NADD Press.

Herman, J (1992). *Trauma and Recovery,* New York, NY: Basic Books.

Hollins, S., & Sinason, V. (2000). Psychotherapy, learning disabilities and trauma: new perspectives. *The British Journal of Psychiatry.* 176, 32-36.

Linehan, M. (1993a). *Cognitive-behavioral treatment of borderline personality disorder.* New York: The Guilford Press.

Linehan, M. (1993b). *Skills training manual for treating borderline personality disorder.* New York: The Guilford Press.

Linehan, M. (2000). Commentary on innovations in Dialectical Behavior Therapy. *Cognitive and Behavioral Practice,* 7, 478-481.

Morasky, R. (2007). Making counseling/therapy intellectually attainable. *NADD Bulletin,* 10(3), 58-62.

Palay, L. (2012). *Autism and trauma: Calming anxious brains.* Columbus, OH: Centre for Systems Change: Disability Policy and Social Welfare.

Poppen, R. (1998). *Behavioral relaxation training and assessment* (2nd ed.) Thousand Oaks, CA: Sage Publications.

Prout, H. T., & Strohmer, D. C. (1994). Issues in counseling and psychotherapy. In D. C. Strohmer & H. T. Prout (Eds.), *Counseling and Psychotherapy with Persons with Mental Retardation and Borderline Intelligence* (pp. 1-21). Brandon, VT: Clinical Psychology Publishing Co., Inc.

Razza, N., & Tomasulo, D. (2005). *Healing trauma: The power of group treatment for people with intellectual disabilities.* Washington, D.C.: American Psychological Association.

Razza, N., Tomasulo, D., & Sobsey, D. (2011). Group psychotherapy for trauma-related disorders in people with intellectual disabilities. *Advances in Mental Health and Intellectual Disabilities. 5*(5), 40-45.

Sequeira, H., Howlin, P., & Hollins, S. (2003). Psychological disturbance associated with sexual abuse in people with learning disabilities: Case-control study. *The British Journal of Psychiatry, 183,* 451-456.

Shapiro, F. (2012). EMDR therapy: An overview of current and future research. *European Review of Applied Psychology, 62,* 193-195..

Sobsey, D. (1994).*Violence and abuse in the lives of people with disabilities: The end of silent acceptance?* Baltimore, MD: Paul H. Brookes Publishing Co.

YAI National Institute for People with Disabilities. (n.d.). Coping: Helping people with DD better cope with their daily problems [DVD/CD-ROM].

White, M. & Epston, D. (1990). *Narrative means to therapeutic ends.* New York: WW Norton.

Wittman, J. P., Strohmer, D. C., & Prout, H. T. (1989). Problems presented by persons of mentally retarded and borderline intelligence in counseling: An exploratory investigation. *Journal of Applied Rehabilitation Counseling, 20,* 8-13.

MODULE VII

Childhood and Adolescence

Slide 1

Module VIII

Childhood and Adolescence

Slide 2

Mental Wellness in Children and Adolescents with Intellectual & Developmental Disabilities

Portions of this module were developed originally by
Phil Smith, Ph.D.
Boggs Center on Developmental Disabilities
Rutgers Robert Wood Johnson Medical School

Mental wellness for youth with IDD and MI has been less fully explored than the phenomenon in adults.

Slide 4

> # Learning Objectives
>
> - Describe issues around development for persons with IDD
> - Describe the stages of typical development for younger children and adolescents
> - Describe how disability effects self-image/self-esteem
> - Describe the key milestones in sexuality and gender identity development
> - Describe the impact of and support around various challenges of maturation

Slide 5

> Childhood and Adolescence
>
> ## Issues of Development
>
> - There is a typical pathway or sequence of development in which certain cognitive, social, and emotional things are seen in each stage for typical people.
> - Functioning and behavior are influenced by stages of development.
> - Intellectual/developmental disabilities often change development due to difficulties in learning, different patterns of interaction, and lack of typical experiences, but most stages still occur (American Academy of Pediatrics, 2013b).

Child development refers to a child's process of learning to do more complex skills as the child gets older. Milestones usually refer to the sets of age-specific skills that children typically acquire by certain ages such as: gross motor skills, fine motor skills, language, cognitive thinking skills (learning, understanding,

There have been many books and materials written for adults, but Baker and Blumberg's book for NADD is the first book entirely dedicated to these questions in youth, and it was not published until 2013. The fact that youth are in schools adds a level of complexity, as there is a dedicated service element for them, but in-home and after-school supports differ in each state and province, and the constellation of services may differ from one community to the next.

One of the significant complexities is that development for typical children is likely to look very different than it does for children with IDD.

Slide 3

> **This module describes issues of typical childhood and adolescence development and details how they are relevant to youth with IDD.**

problem solving, reasoning, and remembering), and social skills (interacting, developing relationships, cooperation, and responding to others' feelings).

Skills such as taking a first step, smiling for the first time, and waving goodbye are called developmental milestones. Children reach milestones in how they play, learn, speak, behave, and move (crawling, walking, etc.).

All children develop at their own pace. However, the developmental milestones give a general idea of the changes to expect as a child gets older. The presence of an intellectual/developmental disability can impact the timeline in which these milestones occur. The delay in reaching milestones, or reaching them much later than the general population, is often the first indication that the child may have an intellectual or developmental disability.

Things which are common in smaller children, such as tantrums, generally fade as development occurs. However, in a child who develops at a slower pace, those changes occur at later ages, which makes it very important to understand the manner in which intellectual/developmental disabilities affects maturation. Is it a tantrum due to delayed emotional maturation, or is it a learned behavior, or is it Impulse Control Disorder?

Slide 6

Childhood and Adolescence

Typical Stages

Approximate ages
- Newborn (ages 0–1 month)
- Infant (ages 1 month – 1 year)
- Toddler (ages 1–3 years)
- Preschooler (ages 4–6years)
- School-aged child (ages 6–13 years)
- Adolescent (ages 13–20)

The American Academy of Pediatrics indicates some of the following as some of the first indicators that a newborn has signs of developmental delay:

Newborn/infant – feeding difficulties, blinking response absent in presence of bright light, poor eye focus or tracking, excessively stiff or loose movements of extremities, does not grasp or hold objects, lower jaw abnormalities, lack of response to loud sounds, does not babble, no smile response (American Academy of Pediatrics, 2013a).

Maturation and movement through stages depends on a wide variety of things, including cognitive changes due to development, physical changes, the presence of enriching environments, and learning through inductive and deductive reasoning. Development also includes the development of a sense of self and identity, which also is impacted by IDD (Black & Baker, 2013). Proper maturation and development of identity is critical for mental wellness.

Slide 7

Childhood and Adolescence

Characteristics of Typical Younger Children

- Often significant issues with attachment and attachment disorders
- Typical developmental tasks related to delaying gratification, task completion, and development of a sense of identify
- Many problems related to impulsiveness and lack of empathy

Attachment is a normal stage of child development and describes the reciprocal, enduring relationship that develops between infant and caregiver/parent. Later development can be influenced by the quality and timing of attachment (Papalia, Olds, & Feldman, 1999).

It is critical for IDD providers to understand what typical children and youth are like. Many things which may be completely typical for a young person can be seen as problem behaviors by an IDD provider who only work with adults. All children need guidance and instructions on these things. What people don't realize is that young people are not just small adults. Working with youth presents an all new type of differential diagnosis: Is this pattern of actions occurring because this person is only 12?

Slide 8

Childhood and Adolescence

Characteristics of Adolescence

Teen life is complex for all young people
- Physically mature
- Sexually mature
- Emotionally mature
  - Desire independence
  - Sense of identity is built
  - Heightened focus on peers
  - Sexual awareness

As with younger children, typical adolescents present an all new type of challenge. Teen years are difficult for all people. It is really interesting that this stage of life is difficult for all people, and conflict and strife are endemic. Efforts to become more adult presents stressors to relationships with care providers. Recall that until very recent times, adolescents were essentially seen as adults. Adoption of adult roles generally occurred in early teen years. The lengthening of childhood through adolescence is a modern occurrence.

During teen years, in a typical teen the person turns from a child into more of an adult. Maturation occurs physically, emotionally, and sexually, and the young person must learn to successfully navigate all of these changes. Parenting and support are critical, and typical forms of parenting and support must be adapted to fit the learning style of the youngster with IDD.

Slide 9

> Childhood and Adolescence
>
> ## Adolescence and Disability
>
> An adolescent with an IDD experiences the same life complexities as other adolescents.
>
> The presence of an IDD or physical disability can make learning and making sense of the world more complex.

These maturational changes may be delayed by physical disability or intellectual/developmental disability that makes learning much harder. Impaired intellectual ability often results in difficulties with inductive and deductive reasoning, which makes it much harder to figure out how the world works.

MODULE VIII

Slide 10

> Childhood and Adolescence
>
> ## Self-image, Self-esteem
>
> - **Central theme – discovering oneself**
>   - Creating a personality
>   - Shaping a personal image of oneself (very self-conscious)
>   - Concerned with outward appearance
>
> - **Often focus on the ways they fail to meet the ideal**
>   - This often results in low self-esteem and unhappiness
>
> - **Shapes how they feel that peers look at them**
> - **Use what one's peers think to determine their self-image**
> - **Try out roles and test these out through social interaction**

Who am I? What am I to do in life? These are two of the central questions in the development of a unique identity. Identity development is among the most important developmental tasks of life, beginning in infancy, but often being resolved during adolescent years. It must be noted that adults also experience a continually forming sense of self. Identity development is never complete. Erikson identified the goal of adolescence as achieving a coherent identity without confusion regarding identity (Erikson, 1959). Identity often is accepted to include physical and sexual identity, occupational goals, religious and cultural beliefs, and ethnic background. The presence of intellectual disability is a relevant aspect as well.

Identity forms through the accumulation of experience and the integration of experiences and interpretations of experience. These experiences begin in infancy when children begin to recognize themselve. Bullock and Lutkenhaus (1990) noted that two-year-olds who see themselves in a mirror with a dot on their nose will then touch their noses. They recognize the image in the mirror as being them, early evidence of the understanding of self. Language use at this age similarly reflects the development of the sense of self, as does representational play (Bullock & Lutkenhaus, 1990). During later childhood, the sense of identity further develops, and often is described in terms of qualities, skills, and characteristics. While this pattern continues into adulthood, where it often includes a focus on various social roles, in younger children the terms are simple, concrete, and unitary; in older children becoming more abstract (Berg, 1999).

Slide 11

> **Childhood and Adolescence**
>
> ## Problems with Self-esteem
>
> Often include:
>
> WHAT MATTERS MOST IS HOW YOU SEE YOURSELF
>
> - Body image
> - Weight problems
> - Shyness
> - Embarrassment
>
> **And for somebody with IDD, awareness of disability.**

The top 4 issues are often true for all people. If I were to ask you what you dislike about yourself, you would have no trouble coming up with a million things. If I asked what you loved about yourself, it would not be nearly as easy, and you might have to stop to think. Our society is very good at helping us know what things are wrong with us and not nearly as good at teaching us to appreciate ourselves for who we are. As adults, we can often keep these things in perspective. We know that advertising is trying to make us feel that we need things to be better or more accepted and loved. We know that movies show people who don't look like most people, being impossibly attractive. Young people haven't yet figured that out in many cases.

This problem is magnified for teens with IDD.

Slide 12

> ### Exercise
>
> Please come up with 10 words that describe you; 10 things that make you who you are.

Slide 13

> Childhood and Adolescence
> ### Risk-taking Behavior
> - **All teenagers take risks as a normal part of growing up.**
> - **Changes in the teen brain make risk-taking more likely**
>   - Time of great opportunity
>   - Risks and problems as well
> - **Taking risks is a tool teens use to define and develop their identity**
> - **Adolescents need to take risks**
>   - Healthy risk-taking can help prevent unhealthy risk-taking
>   - Help create opportunities for healthy risks

Risk-taking is a common part of adolescence for most people. Taking risks can be a way for youth to figure out how the world works and what life is like. The problem lies in youth who take risks that are foolish. We have to teach the distinction between healthy and unhealthy risk taking. That is challenging enough for typical youth, but for youth with IDD it is a greater task. We also have to recognize that for adolescents with IDD, what we might see as a problem behavior may be a manifestation of completely typical teen behavior.

Slide 14

These are the unhealthy kinds of risks. The danger in all of these is evident. In each of these there is a fine line between unhealthy and healthy. We can teach that, but we know that despite the well-known and publicized dangers of tobacco, many, many people still love their cigarettes, chew, and cigars. When does a low-fat diet become anorexia? What is the difference between fudging on taxes and stealing a cell phone? Some of these are exactly the kinds of social judgment calls that people with IDD are notoriously bad at.

Slide 15

Childhood and Adolescence

Healthy Risk-taking

- Sports
- Developing artistic abilities
- Volunteer activities
- Travel
- Making new friends
- Hobbies
- Exploring community

These kinds of risks are the activities that can lead to a sense of mental well-ness, the preventative buffers that can protect us from some kinds of mental health disorders. They reduce stress and improve optimism and well being (Cannon, 1932).

Slide 16

Exercise

- **Identify 2 things you do that are examples of healthy risk taking.**

- **Then think of one negative risk-taking thing you do, but don't write it down or share it.**

Slide 17

Childhood and Adolescence

Supporting Risk Taking

All such activities contain the possibility of failure.

- How can we help provide supports that include realistic goals?
- What skills do young people need to make good choices about taking risks?
- What are some challenges unique to younger individuals?

Failure is a normal part of growing up and a logical outcome of trying anything new. We have to teach youth with IDD to expect failure at times. We also have to teach the reasonable progression of goals from simpler things to more complex things. Nobody learned to hit a baseball with a pitch from a major league pitcher. We learn to swing a bat in t ball. We learn to hit a slow whiffle ball. Trying new things often requires a shaping kind of process.

MODULE VIII

Slide 18

Childhood and Adolescence

Sexuality

- **Key milestones of adolescent development**
  - **Attaining an adult body**
    - **Capable of reproducing**
    - **Intimate relationships**
    - **Complex emotions**
- **Individuals with disabilities may be hindered in this area of development**
  - **Functional limitations**
  - **Social isolation**
    - **Fewer social activities**
    - **Less likely to have intimate relationships**
  - **Lack of information on parenthood, birth control, and STDs**

Walker, Griffiths, Richards, & Dykstra, 2007

Historically, the sexual behaviors of people with an IDD and/or a Mental Illness (MI) have been ignored, prevented, and/or punished by those in charge of their care (Owen & Griffiths, 2009). To explain where we are today, we must examine where we have been.

In the United States and Canada, public perception and professional response to natural sexual behavior in youth and adults with intellectual disabilities and/or mental health disorders have changed over the years. In the early 1900s, sexual behavior of individuals with IDD or MI was seen as immoral and criminal, a scourge on society that must be eradicated through segregation and sterilization.

By the middle of the 20th century, sexual behavior was no longer seen as harmful to society, but harmful to individuals with IDD/MI. During this time, parents and professionals engaged in close monitoring to prevent sexual behavior; education focused on prevention of abuse and exploitation.

The last part of the 1900s focused more on individual rights as an adult sexual being. Because sexuality is such a value-laden and emotionally-charged area, there are still wide variations in how youth and adults with IDD/MI are educated about sexuality; however, service provision today primarily focuses on enabling and nurturing healthy intimate relationships.

Societal attitudes towards sexuality in youth in general present additional challenges for this population. While sexuality has always been a large part of society, instruction on sexuality for youth has been largely a family responsibility in modern western society until very recent times. Sex education and sexuality education for youth depended largely on individual family preferences and mores, and varied widely. In more recent time, such education has been provided by schools and other community institutions and resources, with considerable controversy (Black & Baker, 2013).

Slide 19

Childhood and Adolescence

Development of Sexuality

- Children and adolescents with IDD, like all individuals, are sexual persons
- Most of their behaviors are "typical"
- The problem – often unable to distinguish between behaviors that are publicly and privately appropriate
- Attention to medical, functional, and behavioral issues may shift focus away from addressing sexuality

MODULE VIII

World Health Organization (1976) defined sexual health as: **the integration of the physical, emotional, intellectual, and social aspects of sexual being in ways that are positively enriching, and that enhance personality, communication, and love...every person has a right to receive sexual information and to consider sexual relationships for pleasure as well as for procreation.**

Sexuality develops in persons with IDD in the same manner as persons without IDD. Social judgment in areas of sexuality is a critical concern. Society is often very intolerant of sexual misbehavior, unless one is a politician.

Slide 20

Childhood and Adolescence

Supports

- Avoid judgment and projection of personal values or discomfort
- Ensure the privacy of each child and adolescent
- Promote self-care and social independence among persons with disabilities
- Advocate for appropriate sexuality education
- Help provide knowledge and/or identify a source of information
- Lack of attention to issues of sexuality can lead to misinformation and problem behavior

---

What To Teach
- Teach age-appropriate information.
- Teach appropriate behavior/Teach what TO DO.
- Teach sexuality as personal identity formation and self-awareness
- Teach the right to choose and the right to refuse
- Teach healthy boundaries

Slide 21

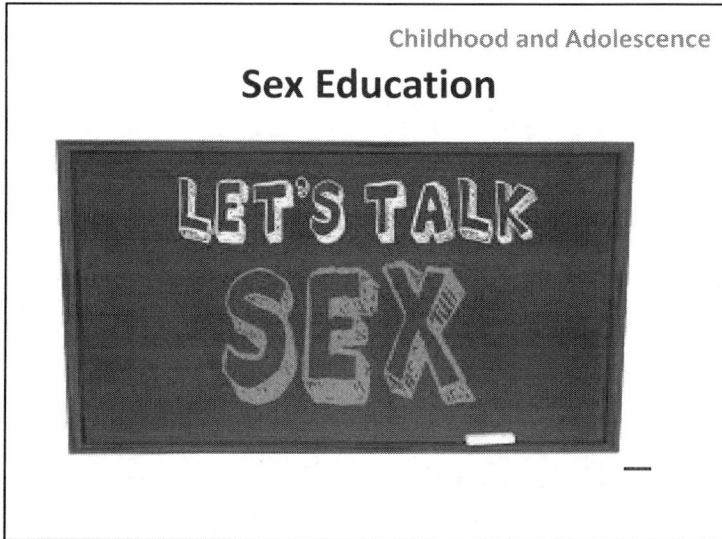

We need to directly teach appropriate ways of telling someone you are interested in getting to know them better. We need to teach how to ask for a date or how to let someone know you'd like the relationship to progress to a deeper level.

Slide 22

In the area of sexuality, professionals often focus on what behavior is inappropriate and what NOT TO DO. The individual with IDD/MI is then filled with ideas about what is wrong, but doesn't understand what behaviors are acceptable and desirable. Instead, we need to teach what TO DO.

Slide 23

Sex and sexuality education often occurs within schools. It is often wholly inadequate to the needs of students in the general population. For students with typical learning profiles, sex and sexuality education need to be more comprehensive and thorough. The needs of students with IDD are even greater. Education in this complex and challenging area must involve all interested stakeholders. Sex education and sexuality education belongs in schools, families, medical or clinical professional visits, and other logical points of contact for youth with disabilities. The question remains, though, does this overly impede the development of a sense of privacy about sexuality? If it is discussed with too many people, overgeneralization may occur and the bus driver may be seen as an appropriate source of sexuality education. Those experiences must be established through careful team involvement and participation.   (Black & Baker, 2013)

It is imperative that the experiences youth have not be "informed" by the media. The media often presents inappropriate examples of sexual behavior, and youth with IDD/MI are vulnerable to seeing those examples as "positive examples" to be emulated. Young people in general have this vulnerability, which has been known since Bandura's Bobo doll research in 1977, and the added complexities of an IDD and a MI make this far more likely to occur. Understanding that popular media is simply entertainment, even when couched as "reality tv," requires abstract thinking which may be difficult for many youth in this target population. Unfortunately, good examples in popular media are few. As such, exposure to media may need to be filtered carefully. (Bandura, Ross, & Ross, 1961)

Slide 24

Childhood and Adolescence

Privacy

- **Teach which behaviors are acceptable only do when they are alone**
  - Provide guidelines about when
  - Review expectations
  - Guidelines about where
  - Ensure the guidelines are followed
- **Identify and recognize cues in the environment (a closed door)**
- **Social cues for public settings**
- **Create cues for alone time (a sign on the door)**

Privacy in sexual behavior is very important. Most typical youth very quickly figure out what is and what is not appropriate to do in front of others. Youth with disabilities are likely to need extra instruction. Especially when one needs assistance in hygiene, personal care does not seem very personal anymore, and privacy can become public. Persons with disabilities can often be treated in dehumanizing ways by well intentioned educators and care providers. This can easily become a problematic pattern. Cues may need to be taught and communication requesting privacy needs to be honored. (Black & Baker, 2013)

Slide 25

Childhood and Adolescence

Working Together

Empower young people to set limits
Assist lower-functioning individuals with achieving & maintaining privacy
When supervising or assisting with personal care:
- Be considerate
- Ask permission
- Remember they still need privacy
- Seek to minimize discomfort

Slide 26

Childhood And Adolescence

Gender Identity Issues

- **In addition to physical development of sexual characteristics, exploration of sexual orientation**
  - Refers to who one is emotionally and physically attracted
    - Heterosexuality
    - Homosexuality
    - Bisexuality

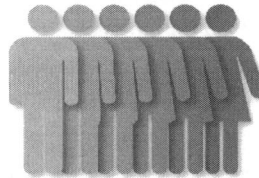

A significant part of a person's identity relates to his or her sexual expression. Alternate choice regarding sexuality is now increasingly accepted and becoming less alternate in many parts of the world. This should be no different for people with IDD, though greater levels of control over sexual expression often result in constrained choices. (Black & Baker, 2013)

Slide 27

Childhood And Adolescence

Gender Identity Issues

Another important task is developing and maintaining intimate relationships

- Physical
- Emotional

Many human rights statements for persons with IDD also call for the full range of choice regarding sexuality being available. This has been a complex issue and is often one of the most difficult areas to address in disability supports. It is relevant to all person, and as society often struggles with expression of sexuality the struggle gets played out in disability supports. (Black & Baker, 2013)

MODULE VIII

Slide 28

Childhood and Adolescence
Peer Pressure

- Peer pressure is one thing that all teens have in common.
  - Need for acceptance, approval, and belonging is vital during the teen years.
  - Teens who feel isolated or rejected are more likely to engage in risky behaviors to fit in with a group
- During adolescence, begin to spend a lot more time with their friends, and less time with their family
  - More susceptible to the influences of their peers

Peer acceptance is incredibly important to all people, but during the teen years, as one tries to forge an identity beyond just being a member of a family, peer acceptance and involvement becomes a greater issue. This has positive sides, but in the case of peer pressure to do things that are wrong or foolishly risky, peer pressure can become a significant concern. The creation of a healthy sense of identity beyond family and peer group has a buffering effect.

Slide 29

Peer Pressure(continued)

- **Pressure isn't always negative**
  - Pressure into negative behaviors
  - Away from positive behaviors
  - Positive influences, such as doing well in school, having respect for others and avoiding taking negative risks
- **Handling peer pressure depends largely on how adolescents feel about themselves**

Learning to handle peer pressure is a part of maturing. Positive role models can provide positive peer pressure. This can be specifically nurtured in young people with IDD.

Slide 30

Bullying

- **Childhood bullies are more likely to become young adult criminals than are non-bullies. Bullied children may grow up with diminished self-confidence**
- **Physical aggression: hitting, kicking, pushing, choking, punching**
- **Verbal aggression: threatening, taunting, teasing, starting rumors, fostering fear, hate speech.**
- **Exclusion from activities**

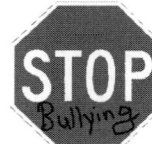

STOP Bullying

M
O
D
U
L
E

V
I
I
I

Bullying is a growing concern world-wide, drawn largely by horrific events. Some countries such as Norway have efforts on a national basis to address bullying; in most of the world it is a local effort, often managed by schools.

Slide 31

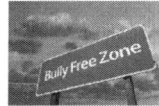

Childhood and Adolescence

Bullying

- Done by someone with more power or social support to someone with less power or social support
- Often includes the abuser blaming the target for the abuse
- Often leads to the target blaming him or herself for the abuse.
- In most bullying situations, the target cannot stop the bullying by his or her own actions.

Many adults who have been bullied remember it is a terrible period in their lives. Youth with IDD are often particularly targeted for bullying due to obvious differences in appearance, skills, or actions and are often seen as being vulnerable by bullies.

M
O
D
U
L
E

V
I
I
I

Slide 32

Exercise

- How do you think the way bullying is portrayed in popular tv shows/movies can affect a young person with IDD?

- What happened and how did the bullying resolve?

Higher rates of bullying experienced by people with IDD can be, at least partially, attributed to societal factors. "Negative attitudes towards people with disabilities go unchallenged as efforts to promote equality through policy are deemed to be insufficiently implemented" (Mepham, 2010).

"[There is still a] prevalent belief that people with intellectual disabilities are not affected by bullying and they do not understand what is happening to them" (Roberts & Hamilton, 2010).

"Early studies on independent living and community based arrangements for people with intellectual disabilities indicated that quality of life is significantly impaired for victims" (Flynn, 1989; Halpern, Close, & Nelson, 1986). People with intellectual disability themselves rate bullying as a leading stressor (Bramston, Fogarty & Cummins, 1999).

MODULE VIII

Slide 33

> Childhood and Adolescence
>
> ### Stop Bullying: What Doesn't Work
>
> 1.**Denial:** ("She would never do that;" "I'm sure he didn't mean to hurt you;" "Boys are just like that;" "Sticks and stones may break bones, but words will never harm")
>
> 2. **Telling the victim to solve the problem:** ("Just make sure you're never alone with that kid;" " Say no;" "Stand up for yourself and hit back ;" "Wear less revealing clothes;" "Pretend it doesn't bother you")
>
> 3. **Broad-brush educational efforts alone:** ("Soft is the heart of a child;" Sensitivity training; "Hands are for helping, not hurting")

None of these strategies work as general interventions despite what Hollywood movies have shown about punching the bully back. If the efforts that the child makes alone will be effective, the need for intervention would not have been raised to this level.

Slide 34

> Childhood and Adolescence
>
> ## Stop Bullying – What Works
>
> • **Consistent enforcement** of effective consequences which are **predictable, inevitable, immediate, and escalating.**
> • **Monitoring** to make sure that consequences and education are effective.
> • Effective **counseling** for youth who bully after enforcement of consequences has generated some anxiety.

These strategies do work and generally require effort beyond what the youngster alone can do. In schools, these interventions are often implemented on a school-wide basis, starting with a national anti-bullying campaign in Norway designed by Dan Olweus.

Slide 35

Childhood and Adolescence

Stop Bullying – What Works
(continued)

- Effective support for targets, including **protection** from repeat victimization.
- **Empowering** bystanders to tell adults, support targets, and **discourage unacceptable behavior.**

Effective support for victims of bullying is important. A culture of non-bullying should be created. This often involves specific instruction about bullying and responses to it.

Slide 36

Childhood and Adolescence

Gangs

- Gang violence has spread to communities throughout the world. In the US, these are the statistics:
  - More than 24,500 different youth gangs around the country,
  - More than 772,500 teens and young adult members
- Teens join gangs for a variety of reasons.
  - Seeking excitement
  - Looking for prestige
  - Protection
  - Make money
  - A sense of belonging
- Few teens are forced to join gangs; most can refuse to join without fear of retaliation

Gang involvement is a particularly risky form of peer involvement, with peer pressure to commit criminal acts being a huge problem. Gang involvement leads to any number of terrible outcomes. Youth with IDD often join gangs as a route to having friends. Gangs can be organized around location, ethnicity, or loyalty. In the United States, gang activity has diminished somewhat from its height, but remains a plague on many communities.

Slide 37

Childhood and Adolescence

Steps to Conflict Resolution

- **Set the stage**. Agree to try to work together to find a solution peacefully, and establish ground rules (e.g., no name-calling, yelling, or interrupting).
- **Gather perspectives**. Each person describes his/her perspective. Listeners pay attention to what the others say they want, and why.
- **Find common interests**. Establish points everyone agrees on. Identify common interests, can be as simple as a shared need to save face.
- **Create options.** Brainstorm possible solutions: both people gain something, think win-win!
- **Evaluate options**. Each teen discusses feelings about solutions. Negotiate to reach a conclusion acceptable to both.
- **Create an agreement.** The teens explicitly state their agreement and may even want to write it down.

Conflict resolution is of critical importance. Conflict between peers can lead to acts of bullying and violence. These six steps are an excellent introduction to conflict resolution. Once again, this framework can and should be taught.

Slide 38

Childhood and Adolescence

Adolescent disorders

- Teens deal with related issues all the time; when it gets out of hand, then it's a disorder
- May manifest differently than with adults
- Common problems:
  - Eating disorders
  - Depression
  - Substance Abuse

MODULE VIII

As discussed earlier, in modern times, adolescents are not just young adults. There are maturational differences, and some mental health disorders presents differently. We will review three of the most common problems.

Slide 39

Childhood and Adolescence

Eating Disorders

- **Anorexia nervosa:**

Intense fear of becoming obese, does not diminish as weight is lost

Disturbed body image – claims to 'feel fat' even when emaciated

Loss of at least 25 percent of original body weight

Refusal to maintain normal body weight

- **Bulimia –**

Recurrent episodes of binge-eating (rapidly consuming large amounts of food in a short time)

often followed by purging – vomiting or laxatives

Eating disorders are dangerous and present significant health risks. Most people want to look attractive. Mainstream media has presented impossible images of what beauty looks like, and young people are at tremendous risk for emulating these ideals. Eating disorders were previously seen as the province of only young women, but young men have begun to evidence increasing rates of eating disorders as well. Eating disorders are often seen as control issues.

Slide 40

Eating Disorders: Causes and Solutions

- Causes
  - Adolescent focus on body image
  - Cultural emphasis on appearances
  - Other unmet emotional needs
- Response
  - Requires formal treatment
  - May include: lectures, group therapy, assertiveness training, drug therapy, and nutritional counseling
- Cautions
  - Avoid arguing, you're not going to talk them out of it
  - Be careful to avoid criticism

Eating disorders must be diagnosed and treated by competent professionals and may require inpatient treatment if the weight loss becomes severe to the point of risking health. Most communities have skilled professionals who are knowledgeable about this. Be careful to not mistake a person who is thin as having an eating disorder. Eating disorders are driven by intense irrational fear, not by a desire to be healthy.

MODULE VIII

Slide 41

> Childhood and Adolescence
>
> ### Early Onset of Mental Illness
>
> - Environmental stress does not cause mental illness, but can trigger onset.
> - Biological events, chemical imbalance or disturbance requires psychiatric treatment.
> - Untreatable mental illness places children at the risk of developing severe forms as adults, more reluctant to seek proper treatment.
> - Poor functioning in school, development, social relationships, family life.
> - Therapy can support, but is insufficient to treat, many severe illness driven symptoms and behaviors.
> - Observation is key to Dx: intensity, frequency, impact.

Early detection of mental illness is very important. Mental health disorders can start in childhood. Effective treatment can follow the diagnosis. Competent mental health professionals can assist in providing the proper supports.

Slide 42

> Childhood and Adolescence
>
> ### Triggers for Emotional Crises
>
> - Onset of illness (medical or mental)
> - Birth of sibling
> - Onset of puberty/adolescence
> - Start or end of school
> - Out of home placement
> - Sex and dating issues
> - Changes in staff & teacher relationships
> - Surpassed by younger siblings or peers
> - Inappropriate expectations of others
> - Physical, sexual, or emotional abuse
> - Illness/aging of parents
> - Death of parent, caretaker, family member
> - Loss of peer or roommate

Any of these triggers should result in observation of a young person to see how the young person manages the stress. Additional support can be placed as a preventative in any of these circumstances. A show of hands regarding each of these that attendees have faced can be illuminating about the number of stressors that typical people face.

Slide 43

Exercise

Consider wellness strategies you can use to support a young person with IDD who might experience one of the emotional crises listed on the previous slide. Discuss with the group.

Slide 44

Childhood and Adolescence

Child Adolescent Depression

- Not just bad moods and occasional sadness
- Serious problem that impacts every aspect of a teen's life
- Requires treatment, can lead to:
  - Problems at home and school
  - Drug abuse
  - Poor adjustment and self-image
  - Negative identity
  - Homicide, violence, or suicide

Depression may manifest very differently in youth as opposed to adults. Depression was not accepted as occurring in youth until fairly recent times. This needs to be considered separately from moodiness that is very common in youth (and adults), and also not confused with labile moods (rapid mood changes). Youth with IDD probably experience depression at a similar rate as typical youth.

Slide 45

Childhood and Adolescence

Depression Signs and Symptoms

- Sadness or hopelessness
- Irritability, anger, or hostility
- Tearfulness or frequent crying
- Withdrawal from friends and family
- Loss of interest in activities
- Changes in eating and sleeping habits
- Restlessness and agitation
- Feelings of worthlessness and guilt

Slide 46

Childhood and Adolescence

Depression Signs and Symptoms
(Continued)

- Lack of enthusiasm and motivation
- Fatigue or lack of energy
- Difficulty concentrating
- Thoughts of death or suicide
- Physical complaints (far more likely in youth than adults)

Which of these are different from adults? The biggest difference is in the physical complaints, such as stomach aches. This symptom is far more common in youth with depression. The technical term somatic complaint is often used for this.

MODULE VIII

Slide 47

Warning Signs, Teen Suicide

- Talking or joking about committing suicide.
- Saying things like, "I'd be better off dead," or "I wish I could disappear forever."
- Speaking positively about death or romanticizing dying ("If I died, people might love me more").
- Writing stories and poems about death or dying.

Suicide is an impulsive act, and youth are more impulsive than adults. This is a significant concern, and any specific worry that a teen might be suicidal or thinking about suicide (suicidal ideation), should be evaluated by a trained professional who will interview the young person and ask a specific set of questions.

Slide 48

Warning Signs, Teen Suicide
(Continued)

- Engaging in reckless behavior or having a lot of accidents resulting in injury.
- Giving away prized possessions.
- Saying goodbye to friends and family in dramatic ways.
- Seeking out weapons, pills, or other ways to kill themselves.

These additional warning signs are of increased concern, of course with the last one being the greatest danger.

Slide 49

Talking Tips for Depressed Teens

- **Offer support**
  - Let them know you're there for them. Avoid asking lots of questions (teens don't like to feel patronized)
  - Make it clear that you're ready and willing to provide whatever support they need
- **Be gentle but persistent**
  - Don't give up if they shut you out
  - Talking about depression can be very tough for teens
  - Be respectful, show you are concerned and willing to listen

These strategies are all important and represent the things that a non-licensed professional can do. We shouldn't always put all of the responsibility on therapists and doctors. All of us can play a very important role in support.

MODULE VIII

Slide 50

> Childhood and Adolescence
>
> ## Talking Tips for Depressed Teens
> ### (Continued)
>
> - **Listen without lecturing**
>   - Resist criticizing or passing judgment; when they talk at least they are communicating
>   - Avoid offering unsolicited advice
> - **Validate feelings**
>   - Don't try to talk them out of depression
>   - Acknowledge the pain and sadness they are feeling
>   - Make them feel like you take their emotions seriously

Listening without lecturing is critical but can be very difficult for adults in helping professions. We want to offer advice and guidance, but sometimes the best thing to do is listen and then validate what the young person says. Validation is important for any person, but particularly a young person with IDD.

Slide 51

> Childhood and Adolescence
>
> ## Substance Abuse
>
> - **Experimenting**
>   - Teens may try alcohol, cigarettes, inhalants, or other drugs one or more times, but not go any further
>   - Usually do not have any problems as a result of substance use
> - **Substance abuse**
>   - Experimenting leads to regular or frequent use
>   - Substance abuse results in problems at home (more arguments), at school (such as failing grades), or with the law
> - **Substance dependence (addiction)**
>   - Physical and/or psychological dependence
>   - Use takes up a significant portion of the teen's activities,
>   - Continues despite causing harm, and is difficult to stop.
>   - An ongoing, and possibly fatal, disease.

Substance abuse is a critical concern for all of humanity. We have become increasingly aware of the damage caused by substance abuse, from car accidents to overdose. Experimenting with substances can be a typical part of adolescence, but that does not mean that we simply accept it. Young people with IDD are vulnerable to making significant mistakes.

Slide 52

Childhood and Adolescence
Health Care

- Adolescents – facilitate a transition to more active role in healthy behavior, medication management, appointments
- Help young people to understand their disability or diagnosis and health concerns
- Identify reliable resources for further information
- Teach healthy lifestyle skills, promote wellness
- Empower them to be more involved in asking questions and making decisions
- Provide guidance in knowing how and when to acquire or decline further help and support

MODULE VIII

One of the tasks of childhood and adolescence is learning to take care of one's health. As a youngster moves into teen years, a more and more active role should be played in this, with the hope of becoming as independent as possible in adulthood. Young people should be specifically taught these items.

Slide 53

> Childhood and Adolescence
> ## Community Safety
>
> - Who/What is dangerous?
>   - Help identify potential danger & make decisions beforehand about safety and trust
>   - Build awareness by reviewing everyday dangers often: fire safety, traffic, crime, internet threats, risk-taking behavior
>   - Build confidence to act safely "in the moment"
>   - Discuss potentially threatening situations
>   - Practice or role play appropriate response
>   - Review who/how to ask for help

The world can be risky. Even in low-crime areas, there are significant risks. In high crime areas, the risks become greater and more pronounced. Instruction on community safety is needed. Everything from crossing the streets to answering a phone can have some element of risk. We need to teach our young people how to safely navigate life so they don't have to live in a bubble.

Slide 54

Childhood and Adolescence
Safety Tips

- Teach the person to always let someone know where he/she is going and for how long
- Routines
  - Many children with IDD depend on routines
  - Avoid routines that others can predict to victimize the kids
- Talk about safety often

SAFETY

These are some general tips regarding safety.

Slide 55

Childhood and Adolescence
Potential Victimization

- Appearance of safety doesn't mean there is no threat

- Grooming– *the establishment of trust through repeated interaction to increase access to a potential victim and decrease likelihood of discovery.*

- Awareness
  - Can children recognize they are being "set-up"?
  - Are parents/care providers able to tell when children don't see it?
  - What "Don't Talk to strangers" means

Victimization is a serious problem for youth with IDD, and adults as well. Recognition of threats and grooming is necessary. Creating an awareness of these kinds of concerns can help, even if they might lead to uncomfortable discussions.

MODULE VIII

Slide 56

Childhood and Adolescence

Internet Safety

- Keep the computer in a high-traffic area
- Establish limits for which online sites children may visit and for how long.
- Remember that Internet technology can be mobile, so make sure to monitor cell phones, gaming devices, and laptops.
- Surf the Internet with your children and let them show you what they like to do online.
- Ask questions about their interests and have them show you what they are searching.
- Bookmark/shortcuts to apps and safe websites for immediate access.
- Continually dialogue with children about online safety.

Young people require a level of supervision with computer and Internet resources to ensure maximum benefit while maintaining safety and security. These are some tips that can be used in a family, classroom, workspace, or residential setting to promote safe habits.

Slide 57

Childhood and Adolescence

Technology Safety

- Know who young people are communicating with online.
- Note numbers of outgoing/ingoing calls with no contact information.
- Open a family/group/house e-mail account to share with younger children.
- Brainstorm screen names and e-mail addresses that do not contain information about gender, identity, or location, and avoid being suggestive.

Some of these tips and strategies are things we can do FOR young people and other are approaches we cooperate on together. Rather than control or isolate teenagers, it's helpful to be involved: validate their activities and relationships and empower them take a role in making sure they are safe.

Slide 58

Childhood and Adolescence

More Technology Safety

- Teach children never to open e-mails from unknown senders and to use settings to block messages from people they do not know.
- Be aware of other ways children may be going online—with cell phones, laptops, or from friends' homes or the library.
- Remind children that anything they send from their phones can be easily forwarded and shared.
- Familiarize yourself with popular acronyms at sites like www.netlingo.com and www.noslang.com/.

Tech safety should be taught. Online activity can lead to less problematic things such as computer viruses, and more problematic things such as victimization. Online bullying has become more of a concern as well.

Slide 59

> Childhood and Adolescence
>
> ## Social Networking: Benefits
>
> **Gain social confidence:** more secure in new situations, such as going to college, joining a sports team, and meeting new friends.
>
> **Learn** about his or her diagnosis and health needs.
>
> **Find support in online communities** – especially true for kids who have unique interests or feel isolated.
>
> **Make friends** who are interested in the same thing or may be dealing with similar issues.

The concerns previously mentioned bear notice, but there are positive things about social networking online as well. Youth from the community of people with Asperger's syndrome in particular have seen great benefit (please note that Asperger's is no longer in the DSM-5, but is still a widely recognized and used term, and we use it here as the community of people with Asperger's syndrome continue to use it).

Slide 60

Social Networking: More Benefits

Keeping in touch with family members that live far away by sharing updates, photos, videos, and messages.

Be Creative sharing ideas or poetry, blogging or journaling.

Increasing media literacy and expand vocabulary and communication skills.

Generates topics for discussion in "live" conversations and with peers in school and other offline settings.

These are all significant benefits that can lead to wellness.

Slide 61

Supporting Young People to Develop Goals

Set realistic expectations – consider:
- Strengths, abilities, and interests
- Opportunities, resources, and feasibility

Be careful not to devalue someone's ambitions

Break larger goals into mini-goals or objectives
- See progress quickly
- Even on a daily basis if needed.

Establish incentives that are meaningful to the person

Be flexible: use setbacks as building blocks to modify goals or create new dreams (turn disappointment into opportunity)

All people need goals. Young people in particular need to have goals. They are often frustrated with not being adults yet, and setting future goals can be of great benefit. Having positive goals also leads to mental wellness. Both small and big goals are beneficial. Sometimes people have goals that others see as being silly or foolish dreams. Telling somebody that their dreams are foolish never seems to help in the long run.

References: Module VIII

American Academy of Pediatrics. (2013a). Age & stages. Retrieved February, 2015, from http://www.healthychildrenorg/English/ages-stages/Pages/default.aspx.

American Academy of Pediatrics. (2013b). Outlook for children with intellectual disabilities. Retrieved February, 2015, from http://www.healthychildren.org/English/health-issues/conditions/developmental-disabilities/Pages/Outlook-for-Children-with-Intellectual-Disabilities.aspx.

Bandura, A., Ross, D., & Ross, S.A. (1961) Transmission of aggression through the imitation of aggressive models. *Journal of Abnormal and Social Psychology.* *63*(3), 575-582.

Berg, L. (1999). Developmental play stages in child identity construction: An interactionist theoretical contribution. *International Journal of Early Childhood,* *31*(1), 11-24.

Black, R.S., & Baker, D.J. (2013). Sexuality and youth with the dual diagnosis of ID/MI. In D. Baker & R. Blumberg (Eds.), *Mental health and wellness supports for youth with IDD* (pp. 83-120). Kingston, NY: NADD Press.

Bramston, P., Fogarty, G., & Cummins, R.A. (1999). The nature of stressors reported by people with intellectual disabilities. *Journal of Applied Social Research in Intellectual Disabilities.* 12, 1-10.

Bullock, M. & Lutkenhaus, P. (1990). Who am I? Self-understanding in toddlers. *Merrill Palmer Quarterly.* *36*(2), 217–238.

Cannon, W B. (1932). *The wisdom of the body.* New York: Norton.

Erikson, E. H. (1959). *Identity and life cycle: selected papers, Psychological issues.* New York: International Universities Press.

Flynn, M., (1989). *Independent living for adults with mental handicap: A place of my own.* Cassell, London.

Halpern, A., Close, W., & Nelson, D., (1986). On My Own: The impact of semi-independent living programs for adults with mental retardation. Baltimore, MD: Paul H Brooks Publishing.

Mepham, S. (2010). Disabled children: the right to feel safe. *Child Care in Practice.* *16*(1), 19-34.

Owens, F., & Griffiths, D. (Eds). (2009). *Challenges to the human rights of persons with intellectual disabilities.* London, U.K: Jessica Kingsley Publishers.

Papalia, D.E., Olds, S.W. & Feldman, R.D. (1999). *A child's world: Infancy through adolescence.* New York: The McGraw Hill Companies, Inc.

Richards, D.A., Watson, S.L. Monger, S., & Rogers, C. (2012). The right to sexuality and relationships (pp. 103-128). In D. Grifiths, F. Owen, & S.L. Watson (Eds.), *The human rights agenda for persons with intellectual disabilities.* Kingston, NY: NADD Press.

MODULE VIII

Roberts, B. & Hamilton, C. (2010). "Out of the darkness into the light". A life story from Ireland. *British Journal of Learning Disabilities*. *38*, 127-132.

Romer, D.(2010). Adolescent risk taking, and impulsivity: implications for brain development. *Developmental Psychobiology, 52*(3), 263-276.

Shelov, S., & Remer Altmann, T. (Eds.). (2009). *Caring for your baby and young child birth to age 5*. Illinois, USA: American Academy of Pediatrics.

Watson, S., Griffiths, D. Richards, D. & Dykstra, L. (2002). Sex education. In D.M. Griffiths, D. Richards, P. Fedoroff, & S.L. Watson (Eds.). *Ethical dilemmas: Sexuality and developmental disability*. Kingston, NY: NADD Press.

World Health Organisation. (1976). Document A29/INFDOCI/1. Geneva, Switzerland.

Aging

Slide 1

> Module IX
>
> Aging

Slide 2

> Mental Wellness and Aging in
>
> People with Intellectual/
>
> Developmental Disabilities

Slide 3

The purpose of this module is to discuss mental wellness among persons with IDD who are aging, considering the experiences of typical persons as well.

Slide 4

Learning Objectives

- Define and describe the components of wellness as it relates to aging
- List the types of changes that occur for people as they age
- Explain the factors affecting people with IDD as they age
- Explain how to enhance supports in consideration of these factors and the IDD
- Describe the age-related health problems attributed to genetically based syndromes
- Describe dementia, the prevalence among people with IDD and the challenges in diagnosing
- Describe the psycho-social aspects of aging with IDD and how to support a person to maintain healthy psycho-social contacts

Slide 5

Traditionally seen as ongoing deterioration and viewed as an undesirable but inevitable end of life process. However, our thinking about the process of aging has changed in recent decades to acknowledge that it does not have to be an inescapable process of cumulative loss of health and function. (Comfort, 1979)

The historical view on aging describes the process with a somewhat negative perspective, inferring that the general quality of health and life of an aging adult is low and suffering is an expected component of aging for all people.

While this may have been and may continue to be true for some people, improvements in health care, economic, and social conditions are changing the experiences of most people as they age. This is particularly true in developed and developing countries. Vulnerabilities still exist but there is now a more concerted focus on disease and injury prevention and wellness in general. Supporting wellness opportunities during this stage in the life span, can enhance quality of life for individuals as they age.

MODULE IX

Slide 6

Aging

Understanding Aging

For some people, the types of changes that occur toward the end of their lives may require more care and support.

As people who have a dual diagnosis age, **understanding and supporting their mental wellness is crucial.**

The process of aging applies to all people, intellectual/developmental disability or not. While many individuals in the general population tend to shift into a "caretaking setting" as they get older, many people with disabilities are already receiving supports under a model of care that can be adapted to changing abilities and needs.

An aging model of care focuses on a group. A disability model of care is person-centered and should maintain that individualized focus as one ages.

Slide 7

> **A New Perspective**
>
> Aging
>
> Clinical definition – "aging is a continuation of the developmental process and is influenced by genetic and other biological factors as well as personal and social circumstances."

Viewed through this lens, aging is a natural biological process that may or may not involve some predisposed health and wellness vulnerabilities.

By assuming that aging will naturally lead to illness, we take on an illness focused approach to disease management as opposed to a preventative approach that focuses on improving all components of health – physical, social, mental.

Ongoing research into prevention of age-related illnesses indicates that the most effective prevention strategy is to focus on improving one's own mental and physical well-being. By being attentive to healthy diet, an active lifestyle, and mental wellness, one can help contribute to prevention of or reduction of severity of age related illnesses.

MODULE IX

Slide 8

> Aging
>
> ### A Diverse Process
>
> The accumulation of changes over time occur at different rates depending on an individual's genetics, environment, and lifestyle.
>
> Physical and physiological changes make the body more susceptible to illness but no certain pathology is predictable without consideration to lifestyle variables. (Saxon et al., 2009)

All people age physically and cognitively in different manners and timeframes. There are actually more "differences in terms of changes and development among older people than among younger people" (Poindexter, 2002). There is great variation from person to person in the processes that occur.

While the prevalence of almost every long term illness (chronic illness) and disability increases and health will naturally decline as people age, sickness is not a mandatory part of growing older whether or not a person has an intellectual/developmental disability (Talarico, 1998).

Slide 9

> # Exercise
>
> **What words come to your mind when you hear the word "aging?"**

Slide 10

> Aging
>
> ### Aging and IDD
>
> Due to factors associated with their disabilities, people with IDD generally have poorer health, greater need for support, and experience greater health-related functional decline than do older people without IDD.
>
> Bir ev. 2004

Many people with IDD experience a combination of disability-related and age-related changes in health. In addition, they can have shortened life expectancy, increased numbers of medical problems, and decreased rates of recommended preventive health interventions.

MODULE IX

Slide 11

> Aging
>
> For some people who have IDD, aging can be complicated by the occurrence of what appears to be premature aging and shortened life expectancy; particularly for people with profound and multiple disabilities and frequently those with Down syndrome.

Life expectancy may also be compromised by previously poor health status and living conditions.

Slide 12

> Aging
>
> ### Aging in the General Population
>
> **Aging in the general population increases vulnerability to certain health issues:**
> - Memory and Alzheimer's disease
> - Sensory problems: Eye and ear conditions
> - Digestive and metabolic disorders
> - Urogenital conditions such as incontinence and prostate cancer
> - Dental conditions such as periodontitis, gingivitis and tooth loss
> - Skin conditions – skin cancers, shingles, dry skin, pruritus, geriatric eczema

Aging is a genetically driven process. Some of the information in our DNA is more likely to manifest towards the end of our lives after decades of environmental influences and lifestyle factors.

Other medical and health-related challenges in one's life can act as risk factors, but there is no blueprint or inevitable roadmap to determine the rate or severity of aging.

In addition to risk factors, there are protective factors that can support the aging process such as: balanced nutrition, activity, hobbies, injury prevention, and social relationships.

Aging is not synonymous with disease. However, the body undergoes lessened reserve capacity during aging. In other words, organ systems are much more easily compromised and take longer to recover from injury or illness. Cell death increases and cell growth slows or stops. Body equilibrium is difficult to restore once it has been lost, causing changes in blood pressure and blood volume, dehydration, and fluctuation of blood sugar.

Health issues identified on this slide are some examples of conditions related to biological aging.

Slide 13

Aging

Concepts in Physical Aging

Skeletal system

Nervous system

Physical abilities are compromised

The skeletal system, including bones and joints, loses mass which can cause osteoporosis, arthritis, bone breakages.

The nervous system -- slows down sensory integration, decreased functional neurons, reduced motor skills, less productive sleep.

Balance, coordination, muscle strength, sight, and hearing are compromised.

Slide 14

Aging

Learning and Memory

Common myths and stereotypes have long implied that older adults are not able to learn new material or that poor memory is part of aging. (Saxon et al., 2009)

People continue to have different learning styles as they age.

Older adults may be cautious about new information or have less opportunity to practice new skills.

Memory refers to ability to recall stored information. But memory also includes how often a person is required to recall specific information.

If one is not required to access certain information frequently or recently, he or she may have difficulty with retrieval.

Slide 15

Aging

Life Expectancy

As a result of advances in health care and community supports, life expectancy is increasing for people who have intellectual/developmental disabilities.

For example, life expectancy for people with Down syndrome has increased dramatically in recent decades - from 25 in 1983 to 60 today.

Several hundred genetic causes of intellectual/developmental disability have been identified and many are yet unknown. The commonality shared by this group is that, individually, each meets the criteria to be considered a person who has an intellectual/developmental disability (based on limitations in cognitive functioning and adaptive functioning).

People with genetically caused IDD may not share commonalities in the way they age or the age-related issues they experience.

Genetic abnormalities frequently cause both cognitive delay and predisposition to specific health issues.

Lack of access to appropriate health services is also an impediment to maintaining good health for a person who has IDD.

While there have been significant advances in research and knowledge about IDD and medical care, many primary care physicians, the gateway to specialized health care, do not have the knowledge or experience to be able to identify the signs and symptoms of declining health in patients who have IDD.

Slide 16

Aging

The Differences in Aging with an IDD

* Genetics
* Environmental Factors and Lifestyle
* Access to specialized health and mental health services for people who have IDD or dual diagnosis
* Communication
* Accelerated aging

Genetic factors that result in both IDD and an increase in specific somatic health problems include a greater tendency to develop upper respiratory problems, early onset of hearing loss, and genetic predispositions to Alzheimer's Disease.

Institutional living and community living both may pose an increased risk of infection, lack of exercise choices, smoking, poor diet, alcohol and drug use, and unsafe sex.

Lack of education about health promotion and prevention can affect diet and exercise. Poor nutrition and obesity are risk factors that can advance aging or lead to secondary chronic illnesses.

People with IDD often have health problems associated with their disability of which a health care provider may not have knowledge.

People who have IDD may not have insight into what they are experiencing as they age. They also may not be able to describe what they are experiencing in a way that others understand. Symptoms can, therefore, go unnoticed until they are more pronounced.

Slide 17

Accelerated Physical Aging

There is evidence that people with IDD develop secondary conditions and diseases. As a result, they may age at a different rate than the general population.

Features of aging that can manifest as a gradual reduction in ability or capacity in an individual in the general population, can occur more rapidly in someone with IDD.

According to Isaacson Kailes (1998), typical aging does not involve a high rate of medical and functioning problems until between ages 70 and 75, people with IDD can show these at higher rates up to 20-25 years earlier.

Sensory changes (hearing, smell, vision, balance, gait) can begin in 40s and 50s with significant limitations in 70s and 80s. For an individual with IDD, he or she may not have coping skills or the ability make behavior modifications to adjust to reduction in acuity and therefore the change is less gradual and appears at an earlier age.

Haverman et al. (2010) reports that people with IDD are at greater risk of health problems that can be prevented. Many of these lead to chronic disease which greatly impact physical health as they age.

MODULE IX

Slide 18

> Aging
>
> **Other age-related health issues are more frequent in people with particular genetically based syndromes.**
>
> - Mitral valve prolapse and musculoskeletal disorders in people with Fragile X syndrome
> - **Scoliosis in people with Prader-Willi syndrome**
> - Recurrent upper respiratory and ear infections in people with Cri du Chat syndrome

Fragile X syndrome is a genetically inherited syndrome that causes an error with the manufacture of a protein the brain requires for normal development and function. It is the most common inherited form of intellectual/developmental disability. It results from a change, or mutation, in a single gene, which can be passed from one generation to the next.

Prader-Willi Syndrome (PWS) is a genetic disorder that is complex in origin but results from an abnormality of the 15th chromosome.

Cri-du-Chat syndrome is a group of symptoms that result from missing a piece of chromosome number 5 and is characterized by IDD. Infants with Cri-du-Chat syndrome have high-pitched cries similar to a cat, which is how the syndrome was named. Most cases of Cri-du-Chat syndrome are not inherited.

Slide 19

Aging

For many intellectual/developmental disabilities with genetic etiology, there are known, existing predispositions for specified medical, mental health, and behavioral challenges.

Mutations in genes that are related to brain activity can cause intellectual/developmental disability. Quite often, these mutations also cause physical abnormalities that lead to health vulnerabilities.

Slide 20

Aging

The most commonly known of these is the increased risk of precocious aging, dementia, and increased sensory loss in people with Down syndrome.

MODULE IX

People who have Down syndrome experience symptoms of aging at an earlier age than the general population. The additional chromosome on pair 21 is known to advance the chronological onset of aging and known to trigger the increase in amyloid precursor protein which is associated with Alzheimer's disease.

Slide 21

> Aging
>
> **The prevalence of certain mental health issues increases with aging, including anxiety, depression, dementia, and psychosis.**
>
> **From the available research, it can be reasonably concluded that people who have IDD are more likely to develop a mental health issue as they age.**
>
> Ref.: Isenberg & Moss, 1993

Although less common than behavioral disorders, major mental disorders still occur in older adults with intellectual/developmental disabilities with an overall prevalence of about 10%. Some disorders, such as dementia, increase with age. Dementia occurs at about the same rate as in the general population, except that it appears at a greater rate (and at a younger age) in adults with Down syndrome. As in the general elderly population, psychotic disorders may also increase with age (although psychoses which appeared in youth may stabilize). They are, however, less frequent than mood and anxiety disorders.

Slide 22

Prevalence of Mental Health Problems

The rate of psychiatric problems for people who have IDD is two to four times the rate of the general population as they age.

The overall prevalence of mental health problems in adults with IDD is higher than in the general population. Factors leading to this higher rate are associated with: higher rates of exposure to traumatic events and/or development of PTSD, lack of coping skills, behavioral phenotypes (psychiatric sequelae of underlying genetic disorders), multiple prescribed medications and drug interactions, repeated pattern of broken relationships, limited choices and opportunities (Royal College of Psychiatrists, 2001).

MODULE IX

Slide 23

Aging

Dementia

The DSM 5 defines dementia as Neurocognitive Disorder. It involves the "loss of memory plus impairment in at least one other cognitive function, such as aphasia, apraxia, agnosia; and disturbance in executive function, which is severe enough to interfere with activities of daily living and represents a decline".

The diagnosis of dementia is made when symptoms have been present for a period (at a minimum 6 months), having ruled out treatable conditions or illnesses.

Dementia presentation may differ between people according to the severity of pre-existing IDD.

Slide 24

> Aging
>
> ### Dementia Prevalence Rate
>
> 22% of adults 40+ who have Down syndrome develop dementia.
>
> The rate increases to 56% for adults 60+.
>
> For individuals with other types of IDD the rate is comparable to that of the general population, 5% in adults 60+.
>
> Janicki & Dalton, 2000, and Fletcher, et al., 2007

Research indicates that the increased prevalence of dementia in people who have Down syndrome is associated with the additional chromosome on pair 21 which can cause increased production of a protein believed to be responsible for the onset and progression of dementia. Nearly all adults who have Down syndrome over 40 years of age develop brain changes consistent with Alzheimer Disease but not all develop significant symptoms (Fletcher et al., 2007).

MODULE IX

Slide 25

Baseline establishment for cognitive functioning and daily living tasks can be difficult for people who have IDD. This complicates measuring changes from baseline to determine if there is a decline in functioning and skills.

Many people who have IDD have difficulty answering questions about memory or higher cognitive functioning which challenges the diagnostic process. As will other health and mental health conditions, limited communication skills and ability to articulate the experience of symptoms complicates diagnosis.

The lack of reliable and standardized diagnostic procedures for dementia complicates diagnosis in the early stages.

A careful assessment of baseline functioning should be obtained, utilizing knowledgeable informants and any written assessments from the past. A continuing data system should be implemented and all observational criteria should be carefully followed and documented.

Slide 26

Case study: Maria is a woman with Down syndrome. She is in her 40s, and her health is failing. She suffers from digestive discomfort and sometimes has trouble hearing. She no longer has the energy to do the things she likes to do, and her favorite TV show, The Office, has gone off the air. Her life just seems to be slipping away. She gets crabby and takes her frustration out on staff, taking an occasional swing when she has energy and spitting at staff when she does not.

Exercise: Think about ways you could use these approaches to develop interventions to support Maria's wellness: Positive Behavior Supports, Mental health interventions, and Person Centered, Planning.

Encourage group participation. Correct answers are not limited to those below; they are listed as suggestions.

Consider the content reviewed in the previous slides and the implications of Maria's age and diagnosis. Evaluate her current health status and advocate for hearing screening and appropriate medical exams/appointments.

Rather than focusing on the TV program itself (reruns, DVDs, other shows etc), identify what elements of the show Maria looked forward to seeing each week that we can possibly replicate for her by finding an "ensemble" community of her own in a part time job, volunteer opportunity or similar setting.

Think about the role that hearing impairment can be playing in behavior challenges and what modifications we can make when addressing her or delivering instruction or information.

Slide 27

Aging

For people who have an intellectual/developmental disability, lifelong attention to preventable medical and mental health conditions is critical for healthy aging.

Health disorders in people with IDD frequently differ from those encountered in the general population in terms of prevalence, age of onset, rate of progression, degree of severity, and presenting manifestations (Sullivan et al., 2011).

Implementation of best practice guidelines in preventative care throughout a person's life span increases the likelihood of healthy aging and the reduction of age-related health and mental health issues.

Evidence-based best practice guidelines for primary care physicians working with people who have an intellectual disability have been developed in Canada. These guidelines include an associated toolkit of information for general practitioners and direct support professionals on general issues in primary care, preventative care checklists, health watch tables and syndrome specific charts, among other resources, etc.   The tools have now been adapted for use in the US health system.

Each of the health watch tables and syndrome specific charts details conditions for which a person has a predisposition and tools for Behavioral and Mental Health.

The tools also include information on how to effectively communicate with a patient who has an IDD.

Slide 28

> **Best Practice Guidelines for Physicians**
>
> Aging
>
> In 2011, Canadian Consensus Guidelines were developed for primary care physicians on evidence-based, best practice in preventative health care for people with IDD.
>
> In 2014. these tools were adapted by Vanderbilt Kennedy University Center for Excellence in Developmental Disabilities for use within the US health care system.

The Vanderbilt Kennedy University Center of Excellence in Developmental Disabilities has collaborated with the Utah Boling Center and the Tennessee Dept. of Intellectual and Developmental Disabilities, funded by Special Hope Foundation, adapting the Canadian Toolkit and guidelines for use within the US health care system. This development provides primary care providers with the knowledge and tools needed to provide comprehensive, preventative health care to people with IDD.

Slide 29

Aging

Primary Care Toolkit

The Canadian Primary Care Guidelines and Toolkit are available at:

http://www.surreyplace.on.ca/primary-care

The primary care tools adapted for use in the US health care system are available at:

http://vkc.mc.vanderbilt.edu/etoolkit/

Slide 30

Aging

The Social Aspects of Aging

As with all people, aging people with IDD deal with a variety of psychosocial changes and support as they age.

* increasing social isolation
* changing interests
* declining energy
* retirement

Continued.....

Jones, 2009

Retirement from employment and or supported leisure activities can have a profound impact on the well being of all people. Transition planning for people with IDD is a critical element of supports to assist in reducing the potential social isolation, loss of income, and boredom that can be experienced in this process.

Supports for people who have IDD should also acknowledge that interests change and energy declines as people age. Social and leisure activities, as well as expectations, should evolve in consideration of the changes a person goes through across their lifespan. Activities for which people have high enthusiasm and interest in their youth may not hold the same appear later in life. Diverse and fluid support plans driven by the needs and wants of the person should be an accepted expectation of people as they age.

Slide 31

Aging

Continued...

* cognitive decline
* financial and estate management
* loss of family and friends
* grief management
* acceptance of mortality
* lack of meaningful work or hobbies

As previously noted, some cognitive decline is an expected outcome of aging. However, it can lead to frustration and declining overall wellness for the person if he or she loses previously achieved life skills.

Aging is associated not only with the increasing likelihood of the death of family members but also with the potential for the loss of knowledge about the past experiences of the person who has IDD.

As with the population generally, the experience of bereavement by people with IDD can be associated with considerable behavioral and emotional changes. When left unacknowledged and unresolved over time, the person will not receive the appropriate support. Loss and grief can also be expressed somatically as symptoms of declining health.

The acceptance of mortality is a healthy part of aging. People with IDD often have little opportunity to participate in the rituals of mortality like funerals and may not have the ability to understand the abstract concept of mortality without these experiences.

Slide 32

Activities and outcomes that enhance social value contribute to mental and physical well being can include:
- Practical, leisure, or life enhancing skills
- Improved or maintained dietary and general health status that prevents physical health factors from hindering typical activity
- A varied rhythm of life
- Recognition that challenge and productivity must continue throughout old age
- An increased and well-established social network
- Participation on a regular basis in the general life of the community with people who are meaningful to the person

Slide 33

Exercise

What social value did you experience from older people as you were growing up?

- **Did you spend time around your grandparents?**
- **Were older people respected during your childhood?**
- **How can we ensure the people with IDD can continue to offer social value as they age?**

Slide 34

Aging

Wellness

Wellness encompasses many components including:

- Promoting health and preventing illness, disease, and injury
- Optimizing mental and physical health
- Managing chronic conditions
- Engaging with life

WHO, 2006.

These four recommendations for healthy aging are identified as those that had the greatest potential for changing or improving the current situation in the area of healthy aging. Focus issues were identified as healthy eating, injury prevention, physical activity, and tobacco cessation (Health Canada, 2002).

Addressing these issues are shared components of wellness for the general and IDD population.

Health care providers serving adults and elders with intellectual/developmental disabilities must recognize that adult and older-age onset medical conditions are common in this population, and may require a high index of suspicion for clinical diagnosis throughout the person's life regardless of the person's ability to accurately self-report.

Slide 35

Aging

Wellness

Key responsibilities for primary care and specialist health services:

1) **Maintenance of the physical and mental health of people with IDD**

and

2) **Early detection and treatment of both physical and mental health problems**

People in the U.S. are living longer than ever before. Many seniors live active and healthy lives. There are things all people can do to stay healthy and active as they age:
- Eat a balanced diet
- Activity for both body and mind
- Don't smoke
- Attend to regular preventative health care and get regular check ups
- Practice safety habits

(NIH: National Institute on Aging, 2007)

Slide 36

> Aging
>
> **Working Together**
>
> As people who have IDD age, there is ongoing need for collaborative supports and services to address the needs of the person in this stage of life to ensure that wellness is assured as an accepted part of aging for this population.

As noted in Module VI – Support Strategies, an interdisciplinary, collaborative system of services is needed for people who have a dual diagnosis across their lifespan, including as they age. There is great necessity for health services, senior services, mental health services and developmental services to make a coordinated effort to bridge service gaps for aging people.

MODULE IX

References: Module IX

American Association of Geriatric Psychiatry.. (2008). *Geriatrics and mental health—the facts.*

Retrieved June 23, 2008 from Available at: http://www.aagponline.org/prof/facts_mh.asp

American Psychiatric Association. (2000). *Diagnostic and statistical manual of mental disorders* (4th ed., text rev.). Washington, DC: Author.

Baxter, H., Lowe, K., Houston, H.,Jones, G, & Felce, D. (2006). Previously unidentified morbidity in patients with intellectual disability. *British Journal of General Practice, 56,* 93-98.

Bigby, C. (2004). *Aging with a lifelong disability: Policy, program and practice issues for professionals.* London: Jessica Kingsley.

Comfort, A. (1979). *The biology of senescence* (3rd ed.). Edinburgh and London: Churchill Livingstone.

Cooper, S.A., (1997). Epidemiology of psychiatric disorders in elderly compared with younger adults with learning disabilities. *The British Journal of Psychiatry. 170,* 375-380.

Fletcher, R., Loschen, E., Stavrakaki, C., & First, M. (Eds.). (2007). *Diagnostic manual – Intellectual disability (DM-ID): A clinical guide for diagnosis of mental disorders in persons with intellectual disability.* Kingston, NY: NADD Press.

Haverman, M., Heller, T, Lee, L., Maaskant, M., Shooshtari, S, & Strydom, A (2010). Major health risks in aging persons with intellectual disabilities: An overview of recent studies. *Journal of Policy and Practice in Intellectual Disabilities, 7(1),* 59-69.

Health Canada. Division of Aging and Seniors. (2002). Dare to Age Well: Workshop on Healthy Aging. Part1: Aging and Health Practices. Works and Government Services, Canada.

Holland, A.J. (2000). Ageing and learning disability. *The British Journal of Psychiatry, 176,* 26-31.

Isaacson Kailes, J. (1998). Dissemination Specialist, Rehabilitation Research and Training Center on Aging with Spinal Cord Injury, Rancho Los Amigos National Rehabilitation Center 7601 East Imperial Highway, Downey, California 90242 http://www.jik.com/awdrtcawd.html

Janicki, M.P., & Dalton, A.J. (*2000*). Prevalence of dementia and impact on intellectual disability services. *Mental Retardation, 38,* 277-289.

Kailes, J.I. (2006). A user's perspective on midlife (ages 18 to 65) aging with disability. (pp 194–204). In: M.J. Field, A.M. Jette, & L. Martin (Eds), *Workshop on disability in America: A new look.* Washington, DC: The National Academies Press.

National Institute of Health. (2007). Global Health and Aging. Washington, DC: Author

Patel, P., Goldberg, D., & Moss, S. (1993). Psychiatric morbidity in older people with moderate and severe learning disability. II: The prevalence study. *The British Journal of Psychiatry, 163*, 481-491.

Poindexter, A. (2002). *Health management of aging adults with mental retardation.* Kingston, NY: The NADD Press.

Ringaert, L., & Watters, C. (2005). The Canadian Centre on Disability Studies Discussion Paper on Seniors with Disabilities. Advancing the Inclusion of Seniors with Disabilities Report (Third edition) for the Office of Disability Issues (ODI).

Royal College of Psychiatrists. (2001). *DC–LD: Diagnostic criteria for psychiatric disorders for use with adults with learning disabilities/mental retardation.* London: Gaskell.

Saxon, S., Etten, M.J., & Perkins, E.A. (2009). *Physical change and aging: A guide for the helping professions* (5th ed.). New York: Springer Publishing Company.

Sullivan, W.F., Berg, J.M., Bradley, E., Cheetham, T., Denton, R., Heng, J., Hennen, B., … McMillan, S. (2011). Primary care of adults with developmental disabilities: Canadian consensus guidelines. *Canadian Family Physician, 57*, 541-53.

Talarico, L.D. (1998). Preventive gerontology: Strategies for optimal aging. *Patient Care, 32*(9), 198-211.

Temkin, M. (2009). *Strategic Issues for Service Agencies.* Victoria, BC: Garth Homer Society.

Torr, J., & Davis, R. (2007). Mental retardation and developmental disorders ageing and mental health problems in people with intellectual disability. *Current Opinion in Psychiatry.* 20(5), 467-471.

Wishart, J.G. (1996). Avoidant learning styles and cognitive development in young children. In Stratford, B., & Gunn, P. (Eds.) *New approaches to Down syndrome (pp.* 173-205).London: Cassell.

World Health Organization (2000). Ageing and Intellectual Disabilities - Improving Longevity and Promoting Healthy Ageing: Summative Report. Geneva, Switzerland: World Health Organization.

MODULE IX

Inter-Systems Collaboration

Slide 1

Module X

Inter-Systems Collaboration

Slide 2

Inter-Systems Collaboration

Peace Bridge,
Niagara Falls
USA/Canada

Slide 3

Learning Objectives

• Articulate how limited collaboration between mental health and IDD systems can result in barriers to service delivery.

• Recognize that assessment of individual need is at the center of effective person-centered service planning for individuals with MI/IDD.

• Explain how communication, cooperative relationships, and knowledge of service delivery are key to supporting someone with IDD/MI.

• Identify the 4 planning and practice elements essential to working together, and the factors that make each of these achievable.

• Describe the purpose, stakeholders, and potential roles of a Dual Diagnosis Committee.

Slide 4

Introduction

• **Barriers to Service Delivery**

• **Principles in Service Planning**

• **Guidelines for Emergency Responders**

• **Community Collaboration and Teamwork**

• **A Framework to Promote Cross System Collaboration**

• **Service Planning Recommendations**

Effective services do not occur in a vacuum but rather as a result of deliberate planning by a variety of stakeholders. At a national, state, or county level there is usually a process of planning that is important and a prerequisite to future implementation.

Although the MH and IDD service systems are the two significant bureaucratic structures, there are usually other systems that need to be addressed in terms of intersystems collaboration. The other systems include for example: education, health, substance abuse, criminal justice, among others.

In this module, we will explore the planning process and provide ideas of how the mechanism of planning can be accomplished.

Slide 5

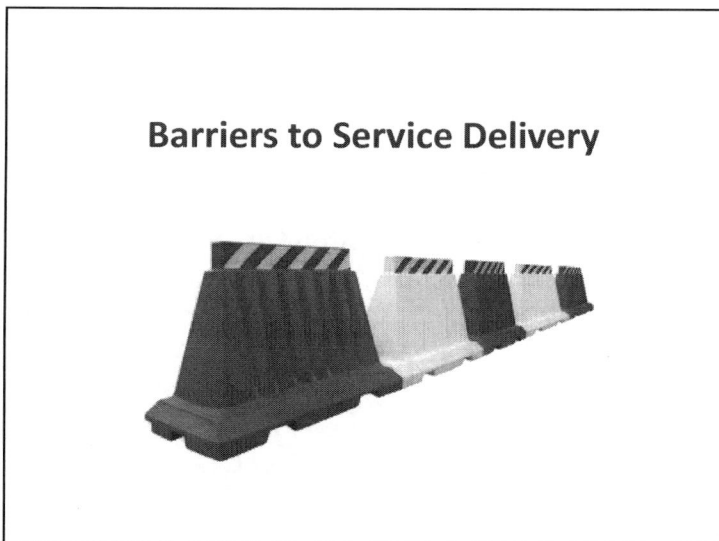

Barriers to Service Delivery

MODULE X

Systems and their related services are often fragmented. Each system is in its own silo. People with IDD who have co-occurring mental health disorders frequently are not understood and do not have their needs met (SAMSA, 2006).

Slide 6

> Dual Diagnosis Policy Barriers
>
> **The Typical Picture:**
>
> **Individuals with MI and IDD are among the most challenging persons served by both MH and IDD Service Delivery Systems.**

Historically people with a dual diagnosis often fall through cracks of the service delivery system, as neither the MH nor DD service delivery system has wanted to take responsibility for their care and treatment (Fletcher 1993 dissertation).

The lack of intersystem planning has resulted in a splintered system of care and has created a quagmire for both the MH and the IDD service delivery systems.

Slide 7

> **Dual Diagnosis Policy Barriers**
>
> ### The Typical Picture:
>
> - **Failure to plan services**
>
> - **Failure to fund flexible services**
>
> - **Failure to obtain technical assistance**

The failure to plan for services for individuals who have IDD and MI has resulted in inadequate care and treatment for this group of people. We live in a 'silo' structure of service delivery. The IDD system lives in its own silo, while the MH system lives in another (SAMHSA, 2006). Each has its own criteria of eligibility, funding streams, as well as policies and regulations. Problems include difficulty negotiating the separate systems (Fletcher, 1993).

The lack of strategic planning has led to challenges faced by states and communities. We have significant systems barriers highlighted by eligibility and access barriers as well as financial challenges (SAMHSA, 2006).

As a result of the failure to strategically plan for appropriate cross-system services, people with a dual diagnosis have not received the services they need. As pointed out "In spite of many innovative developments in service delivery for people with disabilities, success for people with a dual diagnosis has lagged behind that for other groups" (Fletcher, Beasley, & Jacobson, 1999).

Mental health services may be available, but access is frequently difficult for people who have IDD and mental health problems (Mosley, 2010).

There is limited use of medical waivers by states to help address the service needs of persons with co-occurring disorders (SAMHSA, 2006).

Slide 8

> **Dual Diagnosis Policy Barriers**
>
> ## The Typical Picture:
>
> - MH providers perceive that they do not have the skills to serve adults or children with a dual diagnosis.
>
> - IDD providers do not understand the services that the MH sector offers.
>
> - MH providers do not understand the services that the IDD sector offers.

To some extent, policy barriers can be rooted in a lack of understanding of how one system can collaborate with another. Individuals with IDD co-occurring with mental illness are typically supported through different state agencies (Mosley, 2004). Structural differences between the IDD system, on the one hand, and the mental health system, on the other, has resulted in misconceptions and the general lack of understanding of how the two systems can work in a collaborative way.

There is a lack of adequate training for professionals to recognize the possibility of a co-occurring mental health disorder in a person who has IDD (SAMHSA, 2006).

There is a near absence of intersystems professional training and this has led to clinical myths and mistrust.

Slide 9

```
                                    Dual Diagnosis Policy Barriers

    MH System                 IDD System

    · Short term episodic       · Services/supports over
      treatment                   lifetime
    · Focus on psychiatric needs  · Emphasis on direct support
    · Recovery model            · Self Determination
    · Local authority           · State authority
    · Medication Treatment      · Behavioral Support (PBS)
    · Consumer/Client /Patient  · Self – Advocate/ Consumer


        ◄─────────  Little Collaboration  ─────────►
```

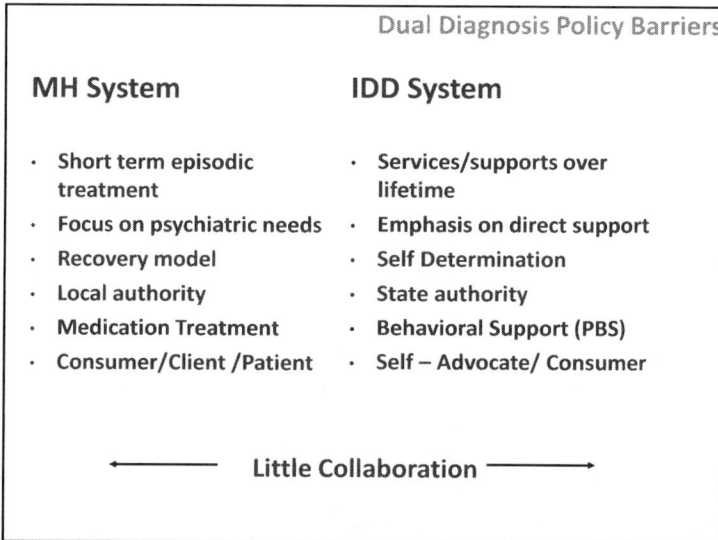

Each service delivery system has its own philosophy of care and treatment approaches. Even the language used in each system can be different than language used in the other system. The professional staff find it difficult to understand and grasp each other's perspective.

Slide 10

```
                Principles & Practices

                          in

            Intersystems Service Planning
```

M
O
D
U
L
E

X

It is important that the systems' stakeholders agree on principles in service planning. The service principles lay out the foundation upon which cross-systems practices can occur.

Slide 11

> **Dual Diagnosis Planning Principles**
>
> - Co-occurring disorders should be treated as multiple primary disorders, in which each disorder receives specific and appropriate services.
> - Collaboration of appropriate services and supports must occur as needs are identified.
> - Services provided to the individual are consistent with what the person wants and what supports are needed.
>
> Fletcher, Beasley, & Jacobson, 1999

The issue of what is the primary vs. the secondary diagnosis has served as an obstacle to service planning and practice. It is important to get beyond this issue in service planning. If a person is receiving treatment services for a mental health disorder, the psychiatric diagnosis is considered primary. If that same person is receiving residential services from an IDD provider, then a developmental disability diagnosis is considered primary for that provider.

MODULE X

Slide 12

> **Dual Diagnosis Planning Principles**
>
> - Services are determined on the basis of comprehensive assessment of the *needs* of each individual.
>
> - Services are based on individual needs and not solely on either MH or IDD diagnosis.
>
> - Emphasize early identification and intervention.
>
> Pritchard, Beasley, & Jacobson 1979

All services need to be based on an assessment of the needs of the person. This assessment needs to consider areas such as mental health issues, developmental needs, health needs, family, etc.

Slide 13

> **Dual Diagnosis Planning Principles**
>
> - Involve the person and family as full partners.
>
> - Coordinate at the system and service delivery level.
>
> Pritchard, Beasley, & Jacobson 1997

MODULE X

The individual and his/her family need to be an integral part of the planning process. Also, the person and family should be empowered to contribute to treatment decisions that are based on a person-centered approach.

Cross systems planning and practice should occur at the systems level (macro) as well as at the service delivery level (micro). Systemic intersystems planning can take place at the county, regional, or state level (macro). The service delivery level involves individual planning at the local level (micro).

Slide 14

> ### Dual Diagnosis Planning Principles
>
> **The system recognizes and values the long-term cost effectiveness of providing best practice services and supports for persons with co-occurring disorders.**
>
> Beasley, Beasley & Goodwin 199?

It is important for the system, including MCO's and other third party payers, to understand the cost effectiveness of providing quality services when needs are identified. Treatment services that are provided by qualified and competent people will lead to positive outcomes. Quality services at the front end will help avoid unnecessary and costly expenses at the back end, i.e., overuse of ER, hospitalizations, incarcerations, and institutionalizations.

Slide 15

> ### Community Collaboration and Teamwork
>
> **Knowledge of Service Systems**
>
> People with IDD and mental health needs are often served by different programs. Treatment and care is enhanced when knowledge and efforts across systems are considered in a community-based approach. This includes:
>
> - knowledge about state and provincial systems and services including education, health care, DD/IDD services, mental health services, inpatient referral process, the justice system, foster care, youth services, community disability services, transportation and employment
>
> - knowledge on issues and practice related to informed consent to protect an individual's confidentiality to promote both privacy and respect for the client
>
> NADD Dual Diagnosis Competence Standards

Collaboration is the vehicle for sharing responsibility, facilitating best practice, and combining knowledge, creativity, and experience of others. The goal of community collaboration and teamwork is building a more effective system for service recipients and greater awareness of the needs of individuals. Community collaboration is often centered on improving access and availability of health and human services, while improving the quality of life for service recipients, and addressing barriers to services (NADD, n.d., Competency Standard 5).

MODULE X

Slide 16

Community Collaboration and Teamwork

Communication with Multiple Systems

Supporting someone with IDD/MI

- Communicate signs and symptoms of individuals' mental health concerns to others across multiple systems.
- Articulate knowledge about the treatment history and current support needs of individuals
- Can present a professional approach to working with others across systems for the benefit of individuals, including sensitivity to the policies and procedures of other professionals
- Can convey complicated information sensitively to others who need to know about an individual's needs and supports, particularly during a behavioral or medical crisis

Effective communication skills are essential and are a key component to presenting a professional approach to working with others across systems. Additionally, he or she must demonstrate empowerment and knowledge, in order to advocate effectively for service recipients. Sharing current and accurate information is the key to obtaining the most appropriate and effective treatment supports.

Slide 17

Community Collaboration and Teamwork

Facilitating Positive and Cooperative Relationships

- Demonstrates ability to navigate recommendations between systems (e.g., psychiatrists and other health professionals, employment, residential settings)
- Demonstrates the ability to build positive and cooperative relationships with other health and mental heath professionals
- Can work positively with multiple systems as a collaborative and cooperative member of the team
- Maintains professional and empathetic communication and partnership with family members and friends of individual
- Recognizes family members as integral partners in support and gathers input from them
- Demonstrates problem solving and teamwork skills

A staff person is often in the position to make contact with and facilitate supports across multiple system, and acts as the liaison between individuals and other professionals providing services. As the main point of contact, that staff person is responsible for providing accurate information, communicating the needs of individuals, and ensuring a collaborative approach to treatment.

MODULE X

Slide 18

Working Together

Effective Planning and Practice Elements

1. **Leadership**

2. **Effective Staff**

3. **Effective Treatment**

4. **Staff Training**

Adapted from Moseley, 2012

Each of these four practice elements is relevant to advance intersystems collaboration. The elements taken together are designed to have a synergistic effect on promoting intersystem collaboration.

Slide 19

Working Together

Effective Planning and Practice Elements

1. **Leadership**
   - **Commitment**
   - **Clear lines of authority**
   - **Commitment to collaboration**
   - **Focus on the Individual**

Adapted from Moseley, 2012

Leadership's embrace of intersystems collaboration is essential. Without leadership to support advancing intersystems collaboration, little can be accomplished from a systemic perspective. Identifying a "champion of the mission," from a leadership position, would facilitate the process leading to a more likely positive outcome.

Slide 20

It is important that the "right" staff be at the intersystems collaboration table. Systems planning requires decision makers who can effectively represent their constituency or system in a manner that seeks to promote intersystem collaboration.

Slide 21

Working Together

Effective Planning and Practice Elements

3. Effective Treatment
- **Appropriate psychiatric diagnosis**
- **Effective medication treatment if needed**
- **Positive behavioral supports**
- **Effective treatment strategies such as DBT, CBT**

Adapted from Mcbride, 2012

Treatment follows diagnosis. Therefore identifying the appropriate diagnosis is crucial. The *DM-ID* (Fletcher et al., 2007) can assist in the diagnostic process. Once a diagnosis has been established, there may be a need for medication. Medication treatment should be aligned with a psychiatric diagnosis. A holistic approach to care and treatment essentially requires both a mental health and a developmental disability approach. Positive behavioral supports should be used along with mental health treatment. Psychotherapy such as DBT and CBT have been growing substantially as they are adopted and applied to people with a dual diagnosis.

Slide 22

Effective Planning and Practice Elements

4. Staff Training

- **DSP**

- **Clinicians**

- **Service Coordinators**

Adapted from Moseley, 2010

Staff training at all levels is a prerequisite to effective planning and practice. At all levels, staff needs knowledge, practice skill, and competency. For example, DSPs need to learn how to observe behaviors that might be indicative of a mental health disorder. Clinicians need to appropriately identify specific psychiatric disorders in persons with limited language skills. Additionally, service coordinators, supervisors, as well as administrators need to know how to negotiate the complexities of various systems.

MODULE X

Slide 23

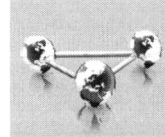

Developing a local, regional, or statewide task force can be very important and useful in the attempt to improve service delivery. The task force can gather information and data to analyze relative strengths and weaknesses in the service delivery system for people with a dual diagnosis. Once there is a clear picture of where service pressures, challenges and gaps exist, a network can build strategies to address them building on the identified strengths to do so where possible.

Slide 24

Inter-Systems Collaboration

Stakeholders from other than MH & IDD systems could be included as appropriate. These include, but are not limited to, representatives from:

- Substance Abuse
- Justice
- Health Department
- Social Services
- Parents
- Consumers
- Advocacy Organizations

- Special Education
- Early Intervention
- Child Welfare
- Coordinated Children's Services
- Service Providers
- Senior Services

The dual diagnosis task force needs to include decision making representation from the MH and IDD systems. The composition of the committee should also include representatives from service providers, family representation, and advocacy organizations.

The working group could include other constituents either on an ongoing or as needed basis. The stakeholders would include, for example, representation from the criminal justice system, special education, and substance abuse.

There is a need for a comprehensive service components to be available, accessible, and appropriate for each individual. This involves an array of service components that need to be coordinated.

MODULE X

Slide 25

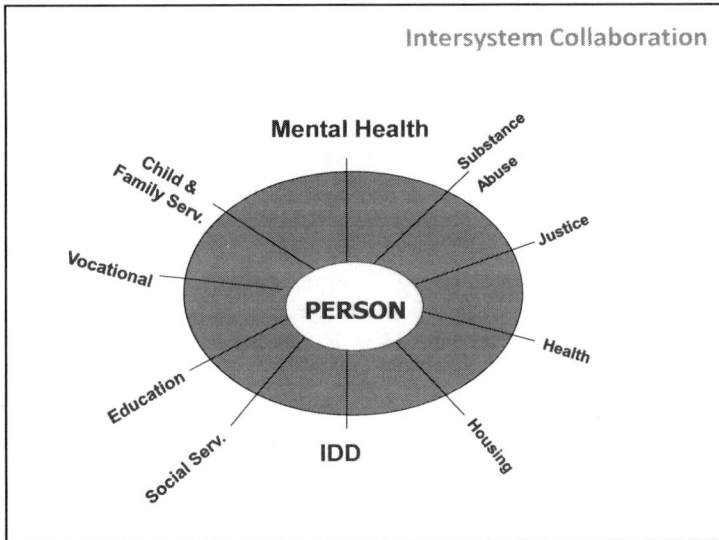

A number of systems need to be involved when it comes to supports, care, and treatment for persons with a dual diagnosis. With the person in the middle, person-centered planning can take place. This would involve an analysis of what the individual wants along with what the individual needs.

Slide 26

This tool can be modified to generate discussion about IDD/MI planning at the local, regional and state level. It is designed to stimulate discussion about "where we are now, and where we want to be."

Slide 27

Tools for Planning

IDD/MI Action Plan

	Action to be Taken	Resources Needed to Complete Action	Date of Expected Completion	Responsibility Person(s) Organization(s)
System Strategies				
State				
Regional				
County				
Staff Training				
Clinical Quality				
Advocacy/ Other				

This is an action plan tool, which can be modified, to articulate the action(s) to be taken. This planning tool should be used after there is sufficient discussion about the issues. It is intended to be a road map of where we are headed with regard to IDD/MI planning.

M
O
D
U
L
E

X

References Module X

Fletcher, R. (1993). *Developing a Policy for the Dually Diagnosed: A Policy Management Model for Providing Mental Health Services to the Mentally Ill-Mentally Retarded (Doctoral dissertation).* The City University of New York: New York.

Fletcher, R., Beasley, J., & Jacobson, J. (1999). Support service systems for people with dual diagnosis in the USA. in N. Bouras, (Ed.), *Psychiatric and behavioural disorders in developmental disabilities and mental retardation.* Cambridge: Cambridge University Press.

Fletcher, R., Loschen, E, Stavrakaki, C, & First, M (Eds). (2007). Diagnostic manual – Intellectual disability: A textbook of diagnosis of mental disorders in persons with intellectual disability. Kingston, NY: NADD Press.

McGilvery, S. & Sweetland, D. (2011). *Intellectual disability and mental health: A training manual in dual diagnosis.* Kingston, N. Y.: NADD Press.

Moseley, C. (2004). *Picking up the pieces of our own mistakes: Supporting people with co-occurring conditions.* Washington, DC: National Association of State Directors of Developmental Disabilities Services.

Moseley, C. (2010). Population based strategies for supporting people with co-occurring mental illness and intellectual/developmental disabilities. Olmstead Policy Academy.

NADD. (n.d.). *The NADD competency-based direct-support professional certification program.* Retrieved February, 2014 from http://acp.thenadd.org/dsp.htm

SAMHSA (2006). Matrix model. SAMHSA's national registry of evidence-based programs and practices. Washingston, DC: Aut

Appendix

Pre- and Post Tests

Module I: What Is a Dual Diagnosis

1. Which of the following diagnostic criteria must NOT be met for a person to be considered to have an Intellectual or Developmental Disability?
    (a) Deficits in Intellectual Functioning
    (b) Inability to work productively at typical speeds
    (c) Deficits in Adaptive Functioning
    (d) Onset of deficits during the developmental period

2. Which of these domains is NOT considered relevant to the diagnosis of an Intellectual or Developmental Disability?
    (a) Vocal domain
    (b) Conceptual domain
    (c) Social domain
    (d) Practical domain

3. Which of these is a common type of Intellectual or Developmental Disability?
    (a) Lovecraft Syndrome
    (b) Zander Disorder
    (c) Aminesis
    (d) Fragile X

4. People with Autism Spectrum Disorder often have difficulties with which of the following?
    (a) Dependence on routine
    (b) Uneven development profiles
    (c) Behavior problems
    (d) All of the above

5. What is a Behavioral Phenotype?
    (a) A type of disability
    (b) A type of mental illness
    (c) A characteristic repertoire associated with a genetic disorder
    (d) A diagnostic code

6. Which of the following does not change when people occasionally experience mental health problems:
    (a) The level of intellectual functioning
    (b) The way they think and understand the world

(c) The way they interrelate with other

(d) The emotions and feelings they experience

7. People with Intellectual or Developmental Disability and Mental Illness:
   (a) Almost never work
   (b) Can only work in a sheltered environment
   (c) Have more difficulty working than the average person with IDD
   (d) Experience very few difficulties in employment

8. Which of the following is NOT a vulnerability for developing psychiatric disorders in persons with IDD?
   (a) Social
   (b) Family
   (c) Psychological
   (d) Vaccinations

9. What of the following is a reasonable percentage of people with Intellectual or Developmental Disability ikely to also have a mental health disorder?
   (a) 0%
   (b) 8%
   (c) 40%
   (d) 80%

10. Which of the following is similar between IDD and MI?
    (a) Intellectual functioning
    (b) Time of onset
    (c) Difficulties in social adjustment
    (d) All of the above.

Module II: Integrated Assessment

1. Which of the following is NOT an example of a medical condition that contributes to problem or maladaptive behavior?
   (a) Diabetes
   (b) Urinary tract infection
   (c) Acid reflux
   (d) None of the above

2. Fill in the blank: The _____ of assessment considers the dynamic influence of four traditional models to arrive at a multi-modal assessment of maladaptive behavior that considers multiple determinants and how each may contribute to the function of behavior.
   (a) Communication Model
   (b) Behavior Model
   (c) Integrative Model
   (d) Medical Model

3. Possible functions of challenging behavior in people with IDD/MI can include:
   (a) To gain attention from others.
   (b) To escape or avoid demands.
   (c) To obtain tangible items or opportunities
   (d) All of the above

4. Best practice in assessment and diagnosis for people with IDD/MI refers to
   (a) The Bio-psychosocial model
   (b) Behavior analysis
   (c) Mental health assessments
   (d) An annual physical completed by a regulated health professional

5. The bio-psychosocial model:
   (a) Incorporates the effects of biomedical and psychological factors and how these influences interrelate.
   (b) Does not require the review of existing data or background information to contribute to the assessment process.

(c) Recognizes that clinical interview can be completed by reviewing the documented history and reports compiled about the person.

(d) Recognizes that mental health is defined only by the relative absence of psychological distress.

6. Which of the premises about people with an IDD is false?

(a) The full range of psychiatric conditions expressed in the general population is also represented in persons with IDD.

(b) Persons with IDD are considered to have a lower prevalence rate of MI than the general population.

(c) Persons with an IDD may tell a clinician or care provider what he or she thinks they want to hear or agree to things to avoid the risk of disapproval.

(d) None of the above.

7. One of the first steps to completing a functional assessment is

(a) Assessing the effectiveness of different approaches on the target behavior

(b) Describing the target behavior; assigning an operational definition.

(c) Identifying the patterns of triggers to help figure out how a behavior is maintained.

(d) Understanding the behavior from the perspective of the person who directly observes it and the problem it causes for other people.

8. The Integrative Model posits that

(a) Problem behaviors can be completely attributed to the existence of a co-existing medical problem.

(b) There are often multiple determinants that influence the expression of maladaptive behavior.

(c) Manipulating the environment in such a way as to increase or decrease problem behavior assists in identifying the needs/ emotions or a person with IDD.

(d) The most effective treatment of problem behavior is teaching communication skills.

9. Which of the following is the most suggestive indicator that a behavior pattern may be the result of a mental illness?
   - (a) The behavior never occurs when the person's favorite direct support professional is supporting him/her.
   - (b) The person appears to be able to start and stop the behavior at will.
   - (c) The behavior is exhibited only at home.
   - *(d) The behavior occurs in all environments; it is not just observed in specific settings.*

10. Which one of the following statements is accurate?
    - (a) Medical problems in people with IDD are easily recognized.
    - (b) Dental problems in people with IDD are easily recognized.
    - (c) Rapid onset in a change in behavior patterns is likely because behavioral problems are directly associated with having the condition of IDD.
    - *(d) Causes of SIB in people with IDD can be related to an underlying medical condition.*

Module III: Mental Health Evaluations

1. Which of the following is an effect of IDD in Clinical presentation?
    (a) Baseline exaggeration
    (b) Eltdown distortion
    (c) Integrative formations
    (d) Crohn's Disease

2. What is the purpose of a Mental Status Exam?
    (a) To measure Intellectual Functioning
    (b) To determine immigration status
    (c) To create a snapshot of the mental status at the time of the assessment
    (d) To make an authoritative diagnosis of mental illness

3. Which of the following is NOT considered in a Mental Status Exam?
    (a) Mood and affect
    (b) Yuggoth's six factors of disability
    (c) Appearance and behavior
    (d) Judgment and insight

4. Who can complete a Mental Status Exam?
    (a) A parent
    (b) A regular education teacher
    (c) An attorney
    (d) A regulated health or mental health professional

5. When might a Mental Status Exam best be performed?
    (a) At an emergency room during an intake
    (b) During an arrest
    (c) Upon being aroused from sedation
    (d) In the middle of a serious behavioral incident

6. Which of the following is NOT a consideration around Intellectual Distortion as related to a Mental Status Exam?
    (a) Inability to label one's own experiences
    (b) Inability to understand common idioms
    (c) Inability to meet ISP goals
    (d) Difficulty describing psychological functioning to others

7. Fill in the blank: Mental Status Exam often must be _____ for persons with IDD
 (a) Ignored
 (b) Modified
 (c) Diluted
 (d) Omitted

8. In assessing General Appearance and Behavior in a Mental Status Exam, a reviewer would NOT consider:
 (a) Terrified facial expression
 (b) Refusal of participation in the interview
 (c) Use of pnakotic language
 (d) Excessive motor activity

9. How might an examiner assess Mood and Affect to a Mental Status Exam?
 (a) Use of Pickman's Model
 (b) Asking the person to use faces to indicate emotions
 (c) Assessing range of motion
 (d) Hazred's Test

10. In assessing Thought Process and Content during a Mental Status Exam, which of the following would least relevant?
 (a) Attire
 (b) Paranoid ideation
 (c) Phobias
 (d) Delusion

Module IV – Signs and Symptoms of Mental Illness

1. The prevalence of depression among adults with IDD is estimated to be:
    - (a) Less than 1%.
    - *(b) 2%*
    - (c) 15%
    - (d) 50%

2. Which of the following is identified as a potential symptom of depression in someone with IDD?
    - (a) Chronic constipation
    - (b) Leaving tasks incomplete
    - *(c) No longer getting up for work/activities*
    - (d) None of the above

3. Which of the following is false?
    - *(a) Bipolar disorder is the most common mental illness among people with IDD.*
    - (b) Borderline personality disorder is treatable.
    - (c) Symptoms of mental illness may present differently among people with IDD.
    - (d) All of the above

4. Type of anxiety disorders listed in the DSM 5 include:
    - (a) Panic disorder
    - (b) Social anxiety disorder
    - (c) Specific phobias
    - *(d) All of the above*

5. The DM ID is helpful because it:
    - (a) It provides a comprehensive overview of the nature of IDD in general.
    - *(b) Includes information on presentation of different mental illness among people with IDD.*
    - (c) Gives the etiology of various mental illnesses
    - (d) None of the above

6. The DM ID offers which of the following in regards to self-mutilation among people with IDD?
   - (a) It is always a symptom of Borderline Personality Disorder
   - (b) It is not a symptom of Borderline Personality Disorder
   - *(c) It can be attributed to different causes*
   - (d)It does not occur frequently enough to be considered

7. Which of the following is NOT a type of Personality Disorder listed in the DSM 5?
   - (a) General Personality Disorder
   - (b) Paranoid Personality Disorder
   - (c) Dependent Personality Disorder
   - *(d) Cyclopean Personality Disorder*

8. Challenges with sleeping due to increased energy, inflated self-esteem, and disorganized speech and increase in vocalizations may be the presentation of Mania in individuals with IDD with a diagnosis of
   - (a) Borderline Personality Disorder
   - (b) Autism
   - *(c) Bipolar Disorder*
   - (d) Schizophrenia

9. What differentiates the anxiety most people feel at different times in life (taking a test, going for a job interview) from anxiety disorders?
   - (a) Whether or not people have an intellectual disability
   - *(b) The amount of impairment anxiety can cause to their everyday lives*
   - (c) If it results in self injury such as skin picking or pinching
   - (d) There is no difference

10. Ruling out medical conditions and considering that "self-talk" may be a learning tool/coping skill for people with IDD are important diagnostic concerns for which disorder?
    - (a) Depression
    - (b) Anxiety
    - (c) Personality Disorders
    - *(d) Psychosis*

APPENDIX

Module V: From DM-ID to DM-ID-2

1. The DM-ID is _____.
    (a) An acronym to describe people with ID
    (b) An organization concerning people with disabilities
    (c) A diagnostic manual for people with disabilities
    A history book on people with ID

2. The DM-ID diagnostic system _____.
    (a) Focuses on the International Classification System (ICD)
    (b) Focuses on comparing the DSM and the ICD diagnostic
       criteria.
    (c) Compares the DSM-5 and DM-ID-2 diagnostic criteria.
    (d) All of the above.

3. _____ refers to the process of over-attributing an individual's
   symptoms to a particular condition.
    (a) Slanted condition
    (b) Aspect concentration
    (c) Diagnostic overshadowing
    (d) Specific review

4. A(n) _____ perspective is emphasized throughout the
   DM-ID to assist the clinician in recognizing psychiatric disorders.
    (a) Developmental
    (b) Reactive
    (c) Aggregation
    (d) Disclosed

5. Psychiatric diagnosis and treatment tends to
    (a) Require a blood test
    (b) Differ only by gender
    (c) Be consistent.
    (d) Vary greatly from person to person

6. Which of the following is <u>NOT</u> a change a clinician should make when
   speaking to an individual with an intellectual disability?
    (a) Ask one simple question at a time
    (b) Wait for the answer before proceeding
    (c) Use music to soothe the individual
    (d) Use visuals

7. In the assessment process, information on individuals with intellectual disabilities should be provided by:
     (a) Multiple sources of information
     (b) Strictly family
     (c) Clinicians/staff only
     (d) Only by the individual

8. _____ denotes a set of behaviors that are genetically determined and are associated with a particular genetic disorder
     (a) Diagnostic overshadowing
     (b) Assessment procedure
     (c) Behavioral phenotype
     (d) Category

9. A particular psychiatric disorder may be manifested differently between:
     (a) Men and woman
     (b) Different seasons
     (c) Different levels of disability (mild/moderate vs. severe/ profound)
     (d) Different income levels

10. Explanatory notes are based on
     (a) Helping doctors keep track of patients
     (b) Breaking down disorders for families to understand
     (c) Separating care providers from staff
     (d) Specific behavior characteristics in persons with IDD

APPENDIX

Chapter VI: Support Strategies

1. People's inappropriate or challenging behaviors are _____; they meet a need or serve a purpose for them.
    (a) functional
    (b) permanent
    (c) evolving
    (d) opportunistic

2. Choose the Components of a Positive Behavior Supports Approach:
    (a) Data collection, physical exam, punishers
    (b) Medication therapy, a behaviorist, positive praise
    (c) Comprehensive data, positive attention, an extinction plan
    (d) Functional assessment, comprehensive intervention, focus on quality of life and wellness

3. Carlos loves going shopping for sneakers but he punches his staff when the store gets too crowed and he wants to leave the store. Considering PBS approaches, choose the best intervention for Carlos:
    (a) Do not allow Carlos to go shopping for sneakers any more
    (b) Pay attention to when the store becomes crowded and be proactive in leaving
    (c) Teach Carlos to ask to leave when he is ready
    (d) B and/or C

4. Which of the following support strategies involves confirming the person's emotions?
    (a) Exploring
    (b) Validating
    (c) Active listening
    (d) All of the above

5. Identify the rational approach to psychopharmacological treatment in individuals with ID/MI:
    (a) Medication can directly affect or stop or control maladaptive behavior
    (b) A psychiatric diagnosis isn't necessary for medication therapy as long as aggression is present

(c) Treatment with medication is used to target the effects of a specific diagnosis

(d) No other supports or accommodations are needed once a person is given the right medication

6. Which of the following accurately describes the guiding principle of Self Determination?

(a) When individuals with IDD have choice and control in their lives they experience increased community integration, as well as increases in adaptive behavior.

(b) When individuals with IDD have choice and control in their lives they experience increased community integration, as well as increases in problem behavior.

(c) When individuals with IDD have choice and control in their lives they experience decreased community integration, as well as increases in problem behavior.

(d) When individuals with IDD have choice and control in their lives they experience increased community integration, as well as more stress and anxiety over choice making.

7. The purpose of _____ is to help the individual self-manage tension and/or anger, and well as distract the person from the source of stress and focus on an appropriate behavior.

(a) Validation

(b) Relaxation

(c) Medication

(d) Choice

8. An effective communication strategy to help deescalate in a positive way includes putting the choice back to the person. What does that entail?

(a) Remind the person that he or she is engaging in an inappropriate behavior

(b) Review for the person the potential consequences if the escalation continues

(c) Remind the person of the more productive and effective choices that can be made

(d) Ask the person to choose how long they are going to take to deescalate

9. Medication complications, inadequate or inappropriate supports, and mental health symptoms are risk factors that contribute to:
    (a) Power struggles and aggression
    (b) People with Dual Diagnosis experiencing a crisis
    (c) Environmental triggers of problem behaviors
    (d) Improved quality of life

10. A crisis plan should include:
    (a) A clear description of what constitutes the crisis for the person
    (b) Clearly outlines actions to be taken by whom at points along the path as crisis unfolds
    (c) Contact information for the resources and people to contact when a crisis occurs
    (d) All of the above

Module VII – Adapted Therapies Pre/Post Test

1. When adapting therapy for a person with IDD/MI, which of the following statements is true.
    (a) The therapist needs to take safety precautions for therapy sessions because a client with IDD/MI will become aggressive.
    (b) The therapist should determine what makes a particular intellectual activity difficult for the person and develop an appropriate adaptation of that activity or use as alternate activity.
    (c) The therapist does not need to address any historical abuse or trauma because people with IDD do not experience hurt or trauma from exploitation or abuse like non-disabled people do.
    (d) The therapist should treat the person with IDD as if they were a child and always use language and techniques used with children.

2. Complete the sentence with the most appropriate response. A person with IDD may seek therapy _____
    (a) For reasons as varied as the reasons for which people without an IDD seek therapy.
    (b) For minor issues. People with IDD do not have the same types of problems that are experienced by people without and IDD.
    (c) When their support staff have thoroughly assessed and diagnosed their maladaptive behavior on the internet.
    (d) When they have the memory retention and self-awareness to participate in traditional, non-adapted models of therapy.

3. Which of the following is false? Whether or not trauma leads to longer term issues and lasting stress can depend on
    (a) The intensity of the stressor
    (b) A person's inherent resilience or vulnerability
    (c) The gender of the person who experienced the trauma
    (d) The time of day the trauma occurred.

4. Complete the sentence with the most appropriate response. Experiences that can lead to longer term trauma for a person with IDD _____

    (a) *Can be related to the buildup of every day stresses and losses that can be unique to their experience.*

    (b) Occur infrequently because people with IDD do not have the ability to experience most situations as traumatic.

    (c) Are not as frequent as they are for the general population due to the limited life experiences of a person with IDD.

    (d) None of the responses are appropriate to complete the sentence.

5. Identify the false statement below.

    (a) CBT (Cognitive Behavior Therapy) has yielded positive results amongst people with IDD.

    (b) The general under-diagnosis of PTSD amongst people who have an IDD leads to a large portion of those with PTSD never receiving treatment.

    (c) Positive identity development can be an effective trauma informed intervention.

    (d) *EMDR is not a recommended treatment for people with IDD who have experienced trauma.*

6. Which of the following statements about Positive Identity Development is false?

    (a) Positive Identity Development refers to one's sense of self that develops through the accumulation of experience, the integration of experiences, and interpretation of experiences.

    (b) Many people with an IDD have a largely negative sense of identity, which is constituted of all the good things the person is not.

    (c) *For a person with IDD, EMDR can be effective in supporting the person to develop a positive sense of self, which can reduce the risk of the person experiencing a traumatic event.*

    (d) All of the above statements are false.

7. Using DBT (Dialectical Behavior Therapy) for trauma treatment, focuses on
    (a) *Mindfulness, emotional regulation, distress tolerance, and interpersonal effectiveness.*
    (b) Integration of both psychological and psychotherapies into a standard set of procedures and clinical protocols.
    (c) Supported positive identity development, mindfulness, distress tolerance and interpersonal effectiveness.
    (d) Skill development and more adaptive cognitive appraisals of events that trigger intense response with strategies presented in a variety of concrete media.

8. CBT (Cognitive Behavior Therapy) is effective in helping improve a person's overall functioning through
    (a) Mindfulness practice
    (b) Engaging subconscious processes and use of archetypal therapy
    (c) Applied Behavior Analytic interventions
    (d) *Skill development and more adaptive cognitive appraisals of events that trigger intense response with strategies presented in a variety of concrete media.*

9. Individual Psychotherapy is most effective for people with IDD when the clinician
    (a) Focuses on increasing distress tolerance through a standard set of procedures and clinical protocols.
    (b) *Adapts a standard technique to the client's cognitive level and engage significant others in the therapeutic process.*
    (c) Focuses on skill development and more adaptive cognitive appraisals of events that trigger intense response with strategies presented in a variety of concrete media.
    (d) None of the above

10. Finish the sentence with the most appropriate response. Group therapy for people with IDD who have experienced trauma_____
    (a) *Helps people foster meaningful relationships, establish a sense of trust, and helps decrease feelings of inadequacy and loneliness.*

(b) Is not beneficial, as people with IDD cannot benefit from insight-oriented group therapy.
(c) Adapts a standard, uniform technique and engages significant others in the therapeutic process.
(d) All of the above

A
P
P
E
N
D
I
X

Module VIII: Childhood and Adolescence

1. Which of the following diagnostic sign is NOT a potential sign of a
   developmental delay in a newborn infant according to the American
   Academy of Pediatrics?
   (a) Reaching for an object
   (b) Lack of response to loud sounds
   (c) No smile response
   (d) Feeding difficulties

2. Which of the following is a purpose of having recognized
   developmental milestones?
   (a) To set instructional expectations for children
   (b) They are a widely used diagnostic tool
   *(c) To give a general idea of the changes to expect as a child
   gets older*
   (d) They have no purpose

3. What is the typical age of a toddler?
   (a) 0 – 1 year
   (b) 1 – 3 years
   (c) 2 – 5 years
   (d) 2 – 7 years

4. Typical children learn how to manage wanting everything
   immediately. The developmental activity associated with this is:
   (a) Attachment to Caregivers
   (b) Developing sense of identity
   (c) Developing empathy
   (d) Delaying gratification

5. Why is sexuality education important for youth with IDD?
   (a) All sexual thought is inherently risky
   (b) Youth with IDD are sexual beings
   (c) They must be protected from all sexual activity
   (d) It is not important

6. Children with IDD are:
   (a) More likely to be bullied than typical youth
   (b) Never bullied because they are always monitored by adults
   (c) Rarely bullied because society doesn't accept it
   (d) Easily taught to stop bullying by teaching martial arts

7. Which of the following is NOT a step in conflict resolution?
    (a) Gathering perspectives
    (b) Threatening violence
    (c) Gathering options
    (d) Creating an agreement

8. Which of the following is a type of healthy risk taking?
    (a) Drug use
    (b) Self-mutilation
    (c) Smoking
    (d) None are

9. Difficulties with self-esteem may include?
    (a) Body image
    (b) Shyness
    (c) Embarrassment
    (d) All of the above

10. Which of the following is a central question in the development of identity?
    (a) Who am I?
    (b) What am I to do in life?
    (c) Both of these questions
    (d) Neither of those questions

Module IX: Aging

1. Due to factors associated with their disabilities, as they age, people with IDD
     (a) Generally have greater need for support and experience greater health-related functional decline than do older people without IDD.
     (b) Generally have decreased numbers of medical problems than the general population.
     (c) Generally experience similar rates of psychiatric problems than the general population.
     (d) Are never able to learn new material.

2. The World Health Organization acknowledges that for people with IDD
     (a) Old age begins at around age 50.
     (b) There is no generally accepted age which defines exactly when people become old.
     (c) Aging is a lifelong process of change.
     (d) b. and c. are correct.

3. Aging, in any population, increases vulnerability to certain health issues. In people with IDD, vulnerability can be increased by
     (a) Genetic factors.
     (b) Institutional living.
     (c) Lack of education about health promotion and prevention.
     (d) All of the above.

4. Age related issues more frequent in people with particular genetically based syndromes can include
     (a) Plantar fasciitis.
     (b) Hypermelatonia
     (c) Musculoskeletal disorders.
     (d) All of the above.

5. As they age, the rate of psychiatric disorders for people who have IDD is
    (a) 2 to 4 times the rate of the general population.
    (b) The same as that of the general population.
    (c) Half that of the general population.
    (d) None of the above.

6. Identify which of the following statements is false. Diagnosing dementia in a person with IDD can be complicated by
    (a) Difficulty the person may experience when answering questions about memory or higher cognitive functioning
    (b) Lack of reliable, standardized diagnostic procedures for dementia.
    (c) Mutations in genes that are related to brain activity.
    (d) Difficulty in establishing baseline for cognitive functioning and daily living tasks.

7. What are key responsibilities for primary care and specialist health services?
    (a) Maintenance of the physical and mental health of people with IDD
    (b) Early detection and treatment of both physical and mental health problems
    (c) Both A and B
    (d) Neither A nor B

8. Which of the following is NOT a possible social aspect of aging?
    (a) Loss of family and friends
    (b) Mental Status Examinations
    (c) Financial and estate management
    (d) Changing interests

9. Which of the following is not a potential component for wellness?
    (a) Optimizing physical health
    (b) Managing chronic conditions
    (c) Promoting health
    (d) None of the above – all are potential components for wellness

A
P
P
E
N
D
I
X

10. Which genetically based syndrome has not been proven to cause age-related health problems?
    (a) Down syndrome
    (b) Fragile X syndrome
    (c) Irritable Bowel syndrome
    (d) Cri-du-Chat syndrome

Module X: Inter-Systems Collaboration

1. People with a dual diagnosis generally _____.
    (a) Easily fit into the ID-DD system
    (b) Easily fit into the MH system
    (c) Can never fit into either system
    (d) Experience difficulty fitting into both systems

2. Services for people with a dual diagnosis need to be _____.
    (a) Based primarily on the mental health concerns
    (b) Based primarily on the level of ID
    (c) Based primarily on a comprehensive assessment
    (d) Based primarily on what services are available

3. Intersystem collaboration means: _____.
    (a) Interacting with your agency colleagues
    (b) Interacting with the person being served
    (c) Interacting with staff from other systems
    (d) Interacting with the individual and his or her family

4. The purpose of a Dual Diagnosis Task Force includes _____.
    *(a) Gathering relevant information to analyze strengths/
        weaknesses*
    (b) Building an international headquarters for people with a dual
        diagnosis
    (c) Using the courts to catalyze change
    (d) Protecting persons with a disability abroad

5. Lack of strategic planning has led to a "silo system" which
    _____.
    (a) Confines people with a dual diagnosis to small areas
    (b) Results in access barriers to required services
    (c) Ensures that people can escape the hustle and bustle of the
        city
    (d) Provides a plan to use state agencies as support

6. The MH and IDD systems _____.
    (a) Always actively collaborate for betterment
    (b) Will collaborate if the person requires treatment
    (c) May work together if the person pursues
    (d) Often do not collaborate, fostering the divide between them

7. Co-occurring disorders should be treated as _____
    (a) *Multiple primary disorders with each requiring active treatment*
    (b) By the severity of the disorder with the more severe being treated first
    (c) By the severity of the disorder with the more mild disorders being dealt with first
    (d) There is no such thing as co-existing disorders

8. The goal of community collaboration is to _____.
    (a) Build a more effective system for individuals
    (b) Raise awareness for individuals within a community
    (c) Improve access to and availability of human services
    (d) *All of the above.*

9. A holistic approach to care and treatment requires
    _____
    (a) A focus on a mental health approach
    (b) A focus primarily on developmental disabilities
    (c) *Both a focus on mental health and developmental disabilities*
    (d) Neither a mental health nor a developmental disabilities approach

10. Systems that are important for people with disabilities
    _____
    (a) Are strictly limited to medical care
    (b) Mostly involve home and family life
    (c) *Should not be limited to any one area*
    (d) Should focus on housing and noting else

A P P E N D I X

Index

I
N
D
E
X

Index

I
N
D
E
X